The *NEW* Hormone Solution

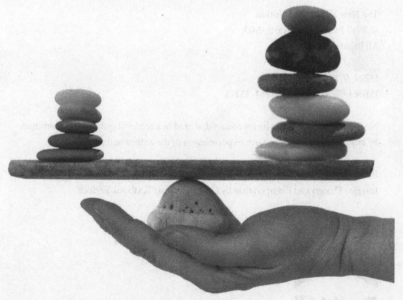

Erika Schwartz, MD

A POST HILL PRESS BOOK

The New Hormone Solution
© 2017 by Erika Schwartz, MD
All Rights Reserved

ISBN: 978-1-68261-330-6
ISBN (eBook): 978-1-68261-331-3

Photos by Gerardo Somozo
Interior Design and Composition by Greg Johnson/Textbook Perfect

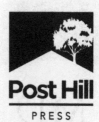

Post Hill Press
posthillpress.com

Published in the United States of America

TABLE OF CONTENTS

This book is dedicated
to all my patients, family, and friends
who believe in my message of health
and who are committed to leading their lives
without intimidation or fear.

To Anthony Ziccardi
and Melissa Peltier

To Lisa, Katie, Jack, Taylor,
Paige, Lucy, and Nellie

FOREWORD

M y book *The Hormone Solution* was published in April 2002. Three months later, the perspective on hormones changed abruptly and dramatically. The Women's Health Initiative (WHI), a large NIH (National Institutes of Health) study on the use of the hormone preparations Premarin and Provera, failed and the use of those artificial hormones was discontinued. As a result, *all hormones* fell out of favor. Premarin, the erstwhile drug of choice for hormone replacement therapy, was banished and more than 7 million women who were taking it (and the doctors who prescribed it) started a long, confusing and divisive process which still continues today. The medical community's "official" recommendations for hormone therapies ranged wildly, from accusing the hormone preparations in the study of causing cancer and completely eliminating them, to integrative, preventive medical recommendations heralding the introduction of natural/bioidentical hormones. Both views have been fraught with controversy; even today, many gynecologists again prescribe Premarin while telling patients that all hormone preparations are the same. Yet both the stories of danger as well as the medical recommendations are based on little scientific information and abound in cover-ups and politics.

The New Hormone Solution is about what happened since then, since 2002, when the entire world of hormone replacement was turned on its head. It offers clarification, details and updates on hormone therapies and their rightful place in prevention, wellness and anti-aging. For the past 15 years, I have compiled the new information for this book, with the help of more than 10,000 patients, and a plethora of research, publications, lectures and clinical research of which I've been privileged to be part of.

The original *The Hormone Solution* opened the door to a then-novel perspective that hormones affect everyone at all ages and that their imbalances can be treated with conventional as well as natural treatments. It also raised awareness of the importance of hormones in health and prevention. *The New Hormone Solution* will offer deeper, more cutting-edge information to help you find the safest and most effective way to add hormones to your medical regimen in wellness and disease prevention, to improve the quality of your life and health. This book will also help eliminate fear and confusion as you try and sort through the confusion and misinformation out there about hormone therapies.

Thank you for taking the time to read it.

and erstwhile progesterone, thyroid, testosterone, thyroid, growth

INTRODUCTION

What Are Natural/Bioidentical/ Human Identical Hormones?

Natural, also known as bioidentical or better yet, human identical hormones, are synthetically manufactured hormone drugs that look identical to the human hormone molecules our bodies make. These hormones are made from soy and yam oils by pharmaceutical processes of concentration and purification that produce hormone powders. These powders are then placed in different preparations for us to take (pills, patches, gels, lozenges, creams, and pellets).

Because these hormones look identical to our own hormones—estradiol, progesterone, testosterone, thyroid, growth hormone, insulin—I believe a better way to identify them is to call them human identical hormones to distinguish them from other hormone molecules that do not look like the hormones our bodies make. Short of human hormones, natural/bioidentical hormones are the closest in molecular structure, actions, and interaction to our own hormones.

All hormones are synthetic because they are made in a lab but if their formula looks like the one of our own hormones they are known as bioidentical or natural in the world of prevention and estradiol, progesterone, testosterone, dessicated thyroid, compounded thyroid, adrenal, and human growth hormone in the conventional world. They are all the same.

Synthetic versus Natural Hormones

Very often you will hear conventional physicians tell you all hormone preparations are synthetic and there is no difference among them. The first part of that statement is correct. All hormone preparations are made in a laboratory. Regardless of whether they are made from plants or raw chemicals they are synthetic, meaning they are man-made. Hormones, unless taken directly out of the human body, are not human.

Synthetic doesn't mean bad. It just refers to the process of creating specific molecules in a laboratory, in this case, hormones.

In the case of bioidentical hormones, they are made from the oils of soy and yams that are plants, thus they were given the name "natural." However, no matter how much soy or yam you eat or slather on your body, it won't turn into the estrogen or progesterone inside your body.

To transform these plant oils into usable hormones we need pharmaceutical manufacturing processes. The products created are fine powders made of hormone molecules identical to the hormones our bodies make: estradiol, progesterone and testosterone. These are what we call bioidentical/natural/human identical hormones.

All hormone preparations are synthetic because they are made in a pharmaceutical laboratory. All hormone preparations do not act the same in the human body.

Bioidentical or human identical hormones are recognized by the human body as our own and no adverse reactions to the hormones occur if when treating humans we follow the individual person's needs for hormones carefully and respectfully.

CHAPTER 1

Why Are Hormones Suddenly Dangerous to Our Lives?

Why is the transition from teen to adult considered exciting and promising, while the transition to menopause portrayed as inglorious and dreaded? Sadly, the truth is that we live in a youth-obsessed society, where wisdom and experience are not held in high regard. For most women, menopause is not a time to feel free or empowered. For most, it represents the harbinger of the inevitable: becoming invisible, less attractive, chronically ill, and old.

As so many of my patients describe it, menopause changes one's sense of self. With both small and large changes taking place every day, week, month, one day you no longer recognize yourself. You give up on the thought that you could ever be your vibrant, youthful self again. Out of 350 million American women, more than 53 million are in menopause today and 33 million will enter menopause in the next decade. That's not exactly a minority. Despite its ubiquitous reality in every woman's life, even in 2016, little serious research on menopause exists. Most physicians are genuinely confused because much of the available information on menopause, hormones, disease prevention, anti-aging and wellness

1

is contradictory and inconsistent, based more on politics and special interests than facts. It is an embarrassment and a tragedy that as a consequence women are still second-class citizens in the 21st century. Our society sends the clear message that menopausal women, no matter how large their numbers, are unimportant. They can no longer bear children, they have lines on their faces and their bodies cannot fit into size 4 clothes. They are invisible at best, irrelevant at worst.

It saddens me that our society hasn't figured out the extraordinary importance of wisdom and experience. We don't seem to grasp the importance of women as advisors and leaders to a better future. Ironically and insidiously, medicine has become one of the biggest culprits in the process of disempowerment of women. Think of the derogatory term "old wives' tales" which fills the medical jargon. Whenever a professor, academician, or senior physician wants to denigrate or discard the relevance of a piece of medical information, the phrase is immediately used to discredit its author. Ironically, after being a physician for the past 40 years, I can attest to the fact that many "old wives' tales" are more likely to be dependable than a lot of the scientifically proven data we bow down to as gospel in the practice of modern-day medicine.

Getting to the Root of the Problem—Hormones

Whether at a dinner, a meeting or a party, all you have to say to a group of women or doctors is "hormones are good for you" and you will start something akin to chaos. Many will announce "hormones cause cancer" or "don't you know about the study that proved hormones are the worst thing you can do for a woman?" Everyone has an opinion and each is dead set that his or her opinion is correct. Passions run high and the conversation becomes harsh and uncomfortable. The more polarized people are, the more confusion reigns. And this confusion will jeopardize your health.

It's high time we eliminate it. Let's get some clarity by starting with the research that started the whole mess.

The Truth about WHI Study

In 1993, the National Institutes of Health (NIH) started an ambitious 10-year prospective double blind placebo-controlled study to compare a specific type of synthetic hormone replacement therapy (Premarin, Prempro, and Provera) with diet, exercise, calcium supplementation, and their effects on cancer, heart disease, and osteoporosis. The results of the study turned out to be catastrophic for women and the doctors who prescribed these medications— mostly internists and gynecologists. On July 9, 2002, the Women's Health Initiative, this particular NIH study, came to an abrupt halt because the data collected revealed increased dangers of heart attacks, strokes, and cancer in the group of women taking the medications. Premarin, Prempro, and Provera were all hormone preparations which weren't bioidentical/human identical.

Sadly, for its impressive size and magnitude, the study was poorly constructed and not representative or applicable to most women who are candidates for hormone therapy. It only addressed one form of HRT (hormone replacement therapy) while other options (bioidentical/human identical hormones) were completely ignored. There were 160,000 women who participated in the study. Of them, 16,000 women were in the hormone arm of the study. These women were, on average, 10 years past menopause, much older than the average woman who starts hormone replacement, and most had preexisting conditions like diabetes, heart disease, and osteoporosis. Many of them were smokers, didn't exercise, or follow what we now consider a healthy diet. The women in the treated group were given the drugs made from pregnant horses' urine (Premarin, Prempro, or Provera); others were given a placebo.

The study was stopped after five years because the interim data (information obtained during the study) showed continuous and significant trending towards increased risk and incidence of heart attacks, stroke, and cancer in the women taking the drugs compared to the women in the placebo group. No other factors that could have caused these women to get sick were considered. Not enough variables or risk factors to determine true connections were looked at in this study. The media made a circus of the outcome and created fear and panic against hormones in general, leaving in its wake doctors afraid of being sued for prescribing the beleaguered drugs and depriving suffering women of the help the drugs provided. The NIH—sponsors of the study—and academic institutions where the study was conducted joined the circus and put out news releases and sent experts out to television and other media with the totally inaccurate and destructive message that *all* hormones are dangerous to women. No scientifically sound data supported their statements. Of note is the fact that the conventional medical societies, such as the American College of Obstetrics and Gynecology and the North American Menopause Society, which designed and executed the study, were receiving significant financial support from the manufacturers of the drugs being studied, Premarin, Prempro, and Provera. These factors instigated a deadly and unnecessary anti-hormone scare that hurt millions of women and confused and splintered the medical profession about hormones as a whole.

Truthfully, the goal of the media tsunami was to take the focus off the true story behind the WHI-NIH study.

Here are the real facts about the WHI:

1. The NIH, a government agency tasked with the protection of the general public health, took money from Wyeth and Upjohn, the manufacturers of Premarin, Prempro, and Provera, and provided free drugs to the academic institutions where the study was conducted.

2. The physicians and researchers who worked on the development and implementation of the study knew that Premarin, Prempro, and Provera were not the only hormone preparations available on the market. There was no scientific basis for the assumption that all hormone preparations behave the same way in the human body. Studying solely one type of hormone preparation was incomplete and the results never applicable to all hormone preparations. *In spite of this fact, the NIH and academic institutions determined to study only one type of hormone drug as representative of all hormone drugs.* Doing so was scientifically wrong and dishonorable. All hormone drugs are not the same, and every class and type of hormone drug acts differently in the human body. What is now known as bioidentical hormones, or estradiol, testosterone, and progesterone, also labeled as natural hormones, were not included in the WHI study.

3. In the wake of the poor results from Premarin, Prempro, and Provera and despite lack of any scientific evidence to the contrary, the NIH and the study's principal investigators at the academic institutions made a calculated decision to bring to the media the story that *all* hormones are bad for women. They feared exposure of the study's great error of omission and that the truth about its bias would emerge, invalidating its results and exposing the special interest connection of the NIH (a government agency) and academic institutions.

4. As a direct consequence, we've witnessed 15 years of fear, confusion, and continuously worsening medical care for women. The misinformation frenzy prompted doctors to take all their female patients off all hormones, "just to be safe." Seven million women stopped taking hormones suddenly, while no one in the medical profession addressed

or even questioned what that sudden, total withdrawal of life-enhancing hormones would do to a woman's body and her quality of life. Tragically, the medical community got their answer anyway even if many are still in denial about it.

The WHI Aftermath

Within weeks after being taken off Premarin, Prempro, or Provera, women started suffering from symptoms often worse than before they had been placed on these hormones. Hot flashes, night sweats, insomnia, loss of libido, itching, allergies, bloating, weight gain, mood swings, depression, and irritability returned with a vengeance. The doctors told women they had no other options as they blindly followed guidelines set by the American College of Obstetrics and Gynecology and North American Menopause Society, now fully on the defensive. Please keep in mind these were the original organizations that made the error of omitting other hormone options to be considered in the WHI study. Instead of acknowledging the error, these organizations insisted on steadfastly holding onto the results of a bad study. This fiasco cost millions of women their health and sanity. These women became just collateral damage of the unhealthy connection among government agencies, academic medicine, and drug companies. Greed took precedence over good patient care.

Time passed and women suffered.

Initially, these organizations disregarded the growing problems the women experienced. Then they provided practitioners with manuals recommending women dress in layers and stay in dark cool places to avoid the symptoms (keep in mind, this wasn't the dark ages—it was in 2003 and 2004!). In time, these organizations recommended doctors start prescribing birth control pills, antidepressants, and sleeping pills to reduce the symptoms of hormone loss to the poor, suffering women.

No woman suffers from deficiencies of birth control pills, anti-depressants, or sleeping pills.

Women Suffer from Hormone Deficiencies

Women do have options. To exercise those options, they need caring doctors who don't simply toe the party line and ignore their patients' needs, but rather develop a solid understanding that menopause is not a death sentence and that hormones are the solution, not the problem. Menopause doesn't happen overnight. It represents another transition in the continuum of changes that make up our lives. Women must become unafraid and confident that the WHI did not define or even partially address the role of hormones in their lives. WHI was a flawed study and its results do not apply to bioidentical/natural/human identical hormones or to hormones in general. The summary of the study from a seminal article in *The New York Times* in 2010 says it all:

Review of W.H.I. Study

SUMMARY
- 16,608 women ages 50–79 (avg. age 63). → Average 13.4 years post-menopause.
- Multi-year study compared synthetic (CEE + MPA) HRT: Premarin, Provera, Prempro vs. placebo.
- Only oral medication were administered (no transdermal).
- Trial ended 2002 (3 years early) due to consistent presence of results linking synthetic HRT to increased risk for CVD, stroke, and VTE.

LIMITATIONS
- Average age of study population was 63 and 10+ years post-menopause.
- Did not include bioidentical hormones.
- Did not include transdermal formulations.
- Did not address confounding factors (advanced age, smoking, chronic illnesses, etc.).
- Results nontransferable to bioidentical hormone therapies (BHRT) or to younger, healthier women.

CONCLUSION
It was clear that the trial had shown physicians something highly important about the perils of starting older postmenopausal women (qualifier No. 1) on pills (No. 2) containing equine estrogens (No. 3) plus MPA (No. 4).

It wasn't the dangers of taking hormones that caused women to stop taking hormones. It was fear and intimidation perpetuated by academic medicine and uninformed, uncaring physicians. It was dishonest information, bad science, and sensational media coverage that created the perfect storm. That can no longer enter the equation when making the decision to take hormones to improve quality of life.

Hormones and the Woman's Lifecycle

Long before we reach the point of being overwhelmed by the symptoms of menopause, long before we feel totally betrayed by our bodies, little by little, one symptom at a time, our bodies prepare us for menopause over the course of more than 30 years. The key to preventing the serious and devastating problems created by menopause is found in understanding the connection between symptoms we experience throughout our lives, and the hormone imbalances causing these symptoms. The symptoms occur from the time we are in our teens and follow us throughout our lives with incredible tenacity. The difference is that at menopause all the symptoms occur at once, causing tremendous confusion, fear, and devastation and our culture often makes a difficult situation worse. Once we stop reacting, we notice these symptoms individually have been present throughout our lives and can easily be traced to our hormones fluctuating over the course of months, days, and decades. Once we connect the symptoms to the type of hormone imbalances causing them—regardless of age—we can treat the problems and prevent them from robbing us of leading healthy and productive lives. In *The New Hormone Solution* I'll provide you with the connections you need to truly understand your body and become knowledgeable and comfortable with the treatments available to minimize the negative impact of the hormone changes you are experiencing. It is my goal to help you feel secure and empowered to make your own decisions. That's what I do with all my patients and it works for them and me. I am sure it will work just as well for you too.

Hormones Awake!

Maybe this is your story, maybe it's your sister's or your friend's. Think back. You are 12. You are an accomplished athlete and a tomboy. You refuse to wear dresses no matter what the occasion. You are not romantically interested in boys, or girls, for that matter. You just want to play sports and follow your friends on FB. Your mother is getting concerned because all her friends' kids are entering puberty and are getting their periods while you show no signs: no breast buds, no perspiration odor, no pubic hair, and, sadly, no period. Fearing something wrong, your mother takes you to the pediatrician. Generic and mostly outdated blood tests (blood count, sugar, cholesterol general profile), a cursory physical examination, x-rays of your bones, ultrasound of your ovaries and uterus, and even CT scan of the brain are all within normal limits. Despondent, your mom is considering taking you to an endocrinologist.

You keep telling her you are fine, but Google and her friends tell her she might be missing something serious. She takes you to the endocrinologist, who does a more in-depth battery of blood tests and tells your mom you could take hormones to speed up the arrival of your puberty. You refuse and your mom goes along. And so it goes until you turn 17. And then, suddenly over a period of six months, you become a woman: you stop being a tomboy, you grow breasts, get pubic hair, start shaving your legs and armpits, you get your period, and start blushing when a boy speaks to you. You just went from tomboy to woman. How amazing.

Or maybe this story is a bit more familiar? You are 28. You just had your third child. The pregnancy was annoying because the obstetrician kept telling you to watch your weight and kept testing your blood for diabetes, which no one in the family ever had. He also sent you for monthly ultrasounds although the fetal measurements (size of the fetus in the womb) were always perfect. You survived being treated like you were suffering with a serious disease during your pregnancy, only to have your labor induced at 41 weeks for some unknown reason (maybe the doctor just had to go to a party or maybe because induction and anesthesia can be billed at higher rates than normal delivery to your insurance carrier). Regardless, you made it through the delivery and your baby is beautiful and healthy.

Although you have plenty of support from your family and friends, six weeks after your baby's birth you find yourself getting depressed. With each passing day, your family helplessly watches you lose interest in the baby and yourself. You finally give in to your husband's pleas to see a doctor. You are diagnosed with postpartum depression. Not that uncommon.

Perhaps you're a little further along, maybe at this stage: You still remember when you were 34 and would come home from work and finally finish with the husband, kids, social media, e-mails, and texts. You were done with another long but rewarding day and couldn't wait to hit the sack. You'd crawl into bed, and fall asleep within a minute. You slept as if you were in a coma.

Not so anymore. Now, 15 years later, you are 47. Your job is secure, your kids have their driver's licenses and are getting ready to go to college, your husband and you have stopped bickering over whose turn it is to take the kids to school, and just when you thought things should be getting easier, life as you know it suddenly changed. It's 10 p.m. You are so exhausted you barely make it through brushing your teeth and applying your five different anti-wrinkle creams guaranteed to take 10 years off your face. You are so tired your bones hurt yet you dread getting into bed because you know what follows will be a torture you were never prepared for.

You fall asleep, but not for long. Suddenly, it feels as though a bolt of lightning has shot through you. You jump up, it's 2 a.m., you're lying in a pool of sweat and your body temperature feels high enough to boil water. The sheets are twisted around you and your heart is pounding. You're no longer afraid you're having a heart attack because the same thing has happened every night for months now, and after two visits to the ER and a complete cardiac work-up you know it's "just perimenopause." You try to ignore this particular episode but then realize you have to pee so badly, you're not sure you can make it to the bathroom. Holding on to the walls, you reach the toilet and pray this activity won't totally wake you up.

You return to bed and pull the blanket to your nose, as the overheated feeling from a few minutes ago suddenly turned you into a freezing mess. You close your eyes and try not to think of the perspiration-soaked sheets, which have now turned to ice. You look around and wonder why the man lying next to you is sleeping soundly, snoring peacefully, while you are such a mess and then become enraged and literally want to strangle him. All you have to look forward to is hours of staring at the ceiling desperately praying you fall back to sleep. Eventually, around 5 a.m. this nightmarish experience ends and you finally fall asleep. Unfortunately, the alarm goes off at 6:30 a.m. and you just want to die. What happened? What has changed between the time you were 34 and 47? What about between 12 and 47?

The answer is very simple: Your hormones have changed.

When we are young, our hormones are in perfect balance and our body produces the correct amounts in the perfect ratios necessary to keep us symptom-free. Sometimes during our teens and 20s we may need a little additional progesterone to help keep the balance at perfect pitch. (More about this later.) When we are young and take birth control pills—which suppress natural hormone production—we suffer from weight gain, mood swings, anxiety, and other symptoms of hormone imbalance. As we get off the pill and start focusing on having children, IVF, IUI, postpartum depression, or just the blues are very common example of hormone imbalances we experience or are induced to have. Still, in our 20s and 30s, significant hormone imbalances are rare and our bodies will rebalance without much outside help, leading to swift recovery. Rare and far between are the women who have heart attacks, cancers, or arthritis in their 20s and 30s without other substantial contributing factors. By our mid-40s, things suddenly start to change. Our hormones (to name just a few: estrogen, progesterone, testosterone, thyroid, adrenals) begin to lose their perfect pitch balance, and we either figure out how to get them back into balance, or we become sick, overweight, unhappy, asexual, sleepless, depressed, and start aging rapidly and getting chronic illnesses.

The New Hormone Solution is here to help you build the deepest understanding of the body you need to create perfect balance for the rest of your life. Hormones are a significant part of fine-tuning that balance—but there are many other ingredients that need to be tweaked, things you must understand that will help you forestall illness, get rid of unwanted symptoms, and restore your energy and vitality at any age.

This may sound like a tall order, but I promise you it is not. Just stay with me and stay focused. I won't waste your time with the medical mumbo jumbo that floods you as you reach out to the internet to learn more about your hormones. I do believe that a clear and simple understanding of the complex physiology of hormones is an important tool to help protect you from making mistakes by following generic advice that may not necessarily apply to you and your needs.

The Hormone Story

Hormones are invisible to the naked eye and that makes them elusive and difficult to understand both to the medical professionals and the lay public. They are produced by specialized cells in specialized organs called endocrine organs—thyroid, pituitary, adrenals, ovaries, testicles, and so on—and they are released and circulate in all body fluids, directly affecting the activity of every cell in every organ in our body. Hormones may stimulate or suppress the actions of organs and their individual cells everywhere in the body. No organ is left untouched by the actions of hormones.

When It Comes to Prevention, Endocrinology Is Totally Out of Touch

Even though endocrinology is considered a subspecialty that deals with hormones, the field is sadly outdated and doesn't help patients before diseases set in. Conventional endocrinologists are trained to search for disease by doing exhaustive tests, and then just putting a label on the patient accordingly. Many patients I see spend years seeing endocrinologists and still their thyroid function is out of balance because the doctor is treating blood result numbers and not patients. Symptoms are ignored because doctors do not believe or understand the patient is what matters, not the numbers on a blood tests. The doctors are also clueless about true prevention. No medical or post graduate education exists in the field. This leaves the entire area of hormone balance in wellness and disease prevention to the group of doctors I belong to—a new breed who, while conventionally trained, remember the answers lie with the patients and their symptoms, and not the numbers on blood tests. This new breed of doctors focuses on prevention and listens, cares, and treats the whole patient, not blood results or individual organ systems.

Why Are Hormones So Important Anyway?

As our hormones travel to every cell in our bodies they affect every organ and cell function on their way. From the ways we breathe, think, digest, move, sleep, exercise, make love, everything humans do is hormone-driven. Hormones have the power to make us feel great or ruin our lives. There are myriad of hormones with very important functions.

Let's start with the sex hormones: estrogen, progesterone, and testosterone. They don't just determine our gender and how interested we are in having sex or building muscle, they are responsible for our outlook and reactions in life, how we age, and how long we live. (For more about the physiology of hormones, please see Appendices A and B.)

Estrogen, Progesterone, and Testosterone— the Sex Hormones

There are many sex hormone-like drugs (substances that fool our bodies into thinking they are sex hormones); birth control pills are a perfect example. They are drugs that are created to fit into certain hormone receptors in the walls of our cells. They are like round pegs trying to fit into square holes. They don't quite fit but the body makes do with them; their actions specifically address one hormone action and their side-effects produce hundreds of undesirable problems. Drug companies are in the business of making these drugs because they can be patented and they can obtain FDA approval for their use. For example: birth control pills prevent ovulation, medroxyprogesterone acetate (Provera) counteracts a negative side-effect—thickening the uterine lining associated with conjugated equine estrogen (Premarin). Tamoxifen blocks estrogen effect in the body. Premarin may treat vaginal atrophy. Others, like Brisdelle, an antidepressant specifically used to treat hot flashes, are SSRIs (selective serotonin reuptake inhibitors). Addyi, another antidepressant derivative, is FDA-approved to improve sex drive. While these drugs come with specific FDA-approved indications, they have side-effects, often suppressing the natural action of our own sex hormones, at times leaving us depleted, infertile, and sick. While the side-effects are explicitly explained in the pamphlets included with the drug, most doctors won't tell you about them, nor is it likely you will read the extensive small print in the package insert. That is not an error of commission, it is simply too long and every FDA-approved drug lists every possible side-effect associated with it. That is because drugs are substances foreign to the human body that may treat one particular symptom but are guaranteed to create other, often unexpected, symptoms.

As of 2016, there are only three *real* human end-organ (ovary and testicle) sex hormones known: estrogen, progesterone, and testosterone. Both men and women have all three. The difference between men and women lies in the amounts of these hormones circulating in our bloodstreams.

Estrogen is the dominant hormone in women. The dominant hormone in men is testosterone.

A significant shortcoming in our understanding of hormones is the belief that estrogen, progesterone, and testosterone act independently of one another. Unless we totally incorporate into our understanding their inseparability and interconnection, we cannot effectively or safely solve the problems caused by imbalances or depletion in their individual levels.

Hormones are intimately involved in every body function. The amount of hormones secreted are controlled by two glands in the brain—the hypothalamus and the pituitary. Sex hormones are produced primarily by the sex organs: ovaries, testicles, and the adrenal glands. There are three major sex hormones: estrogen, progesterone, and testosterone. Their actions are interconnected and are both positive and negative. The balance and interaction among sex hormones define the presence or absence of symptoms, health or disease.

For more details please read Appendix A, "Physiology of Hormones" and Appendix B, "Sex Hormones 101."

In the chapters that follow, I promise you insights that will change your life for the better and bring clarity and focus, eliminate any fear of hormones, and empower you to lead healthier, happier, and balanced lives.

16

CHAPTER 2

The Theory of Hormones

Hormones Determine Gender Characteristics: Male or Female

Now that we've gotten the scientific 101 on sex hormones, their production, and interrelation, let's see how they affect our lives at various ages and under different circumstances.

Physical differences between males and females appear early in the development of the fetus in the uterus. As the fertilized egg is implanted into the soft, warm lining of the uterus, hormone levels skyrocket. By the time the first or second ultrasound is taken of the fetus in the womb, between 16 to 20 weeks, the difference in sexes is clearly visible. High, well-balanced levels of sex hormones in the mother are mandatory for the survival and growth of the fetus. But once the baby is born and no longer has access to the mom's hormones, sexual differentiation comes to a screeching halt. For the following 10 to 12 years (with the exception of early puberty, which is a topic by itself), the difference between boys and girls is purely cultural and sociologic. Breasts don't sprout, penises don't grow, young children are sexually dormant.

What is going on here?

Our marvelous sex hormones have decided to take a break. They have gone into a hibernation phase while the baby grows from a newborn to toddler to young child. It's time for the body to focus on other things. Growth of the body organs, development of the brain and muscle coordination take precedence over development of sexual characteristics. This nonsexual focus is actually a saving grace and a blessing. Consider the confusion early puberty creates in young children and those surrounding them. Researchers are still trying to untangle the meaning of the increasing incidence of early sexual development in 7- to 10-year-old girls and boys—not easy to understand even if environmental factors may be at fault. We still have to deal with these dramatic changes. Not only is this development worrisome from the physiologic standpoint, it has enormous psychological impact. We desperately need the dormancy period to properly develop and mature physically and emotionally before we become sexual beings. This lag time is tantamount to normal development of a human being. Anatomic and emotional maturation are critical and need time. If that time is not given, both boys and girls are in danger of never being able to mature emotionally because the wallop of sex hormones affects human behavior permanently once it declares itself.

At puberty—for most this occurs between the ages of 10 to 13—the sleepy sex hormones suddenly wake up. The sex glands—testes, ovaries, and part of the adrenals—start making up for lost time and manufacture copious amounts of sex hormones. Estrogen, progesterone, and testosterone are flooding the system. The rapid transformation from girl to woman and from boy to man is like a tsunami; it overtakes everything in its way.

From Girl to Woman

For most people, increasing levels of estrogen, progesterone, and testosterone translate into the emergence of a young adult.

In medical terms this change is referred to as the appearance of secondary sex characteristics.

During middle school, when your children undergo maturity physicals, a doctor looks for the appearance of these secondary sexual characteristics to determine your child's stage of physical maturation. While to the naked eye we see growing breasts, pubic and armpit hair, and adult-smelling perspiration, few of us consciously realize these are outward signs of sex hormones working inside the young child's body.

The girl starts to have a period and also may ovulate (release an egg). By the time girls are in their early 20s, periods are pretty much monthly occurrences and ovulation becomes regular. Physiologically this means the girl is physically ready to have children of her own. Irregular periods and ovulations are normal into the 20s and any concern about regulating periods with birth control pills is not based on any scientific fact but rather is a marketing ploy to sell more birth control pills. The cavalier birth control-prescribing practices of gynecologists is a direct consequence of their training sponsored by special interest groups and is not based on human physiology.

From Boy to Man

Boys follow the same path.

Who hasn't heard the cracking voice of a 12-year old boy turned from soprano to frog to baritone overnight? And how remarkable is the sudden appearance of facial hair and the growth spurt that turns your little boy into a towering man? The acne and change in behavior are also part and parcel of the fingerprint sex hormones leave in their wake. What we don't connect so readily is that the same hormones have induced the growth of pubic hair, body odor and enlargement of the penis and testicles. And these changes address only the impact hormones have on physical development.

How about the behavioral changes directly connected to the impact of hormones; the suddenly sullen, unwilling-to-communicate teen who slams the door shut to his bedroom in your face is the same little boy who only a few months ago held tightly onto your hand while crossing the street. To parents the transition is remarkable and often difficult to accept.

Studies have shown that although environment and culture have significant impacts on our general outlook, it is the sex hormones that direct women to become nesters, desirous of having babies, while men focus on sports, physical activities, competitive endeavors, and, of course, sex. This is a critical moment in the development of our species. Hormones impact the pubescent child, culture steers behavior, and society predetermines the acceptable roles for males and females.

Children who suffer from hormone deficiency syndromes or genetic XY chromosome differences (Turner (45X) and Klinefelter (47XXY) syndromes) maintain a sexually neutral attitude in life. They do not exhibit either male- or female-specific emotional and often physical traits. The typical asexual he/she we encounter in comedies and in our everyday lives are perfect examples of human beings not responding to the influence of sex hormones. Some call them asexual, some think these people don't really exist, and some think they are homosexual and unable or unwilling to express their gender identity; but truth is, they are just humans who may be genetically similar to the majority, yet they invariably are low in or insensitive to the impact of sex hormones.

How Hormones Keep Mankind from Becoming an Endangered Species

During the first 8 to 10 years of life our sex hormones are in hibernation. They are preparing for their moment in the spotlight, the moment we recognize as puberty and then adolescence.

Teenagers

The term "adolescence" doesn't quite explain why the sweet 8-year-old who only yesterday cuddled and told you, "I love you, Mommy" suddenly wakes up at the age of 11, having decided that you are a moron and an embarrassment. The term adolescence just gives us a label for inexplicable and often intolerable behavior. There is a critical but physiologic reason for the irrationality and speed of the transition from puberty to adolescent behavior. In our culture, we glibly call it "hormone storm."

For years, parents have justified their teen and even tween son's or daughter's unreasonable and often rude behavior with the catchall phrase "it's their hormones." The only problem is that when we refer to this so-called "hormone storm," we think of their irrational behavior in terms of overflowing sexuality. We clearly attribute teenagers' pimples and their short fuses to parental advice to hormones, but we fail to realize another more significant effect hormones have on our teens.

We rarely notice how incredibly healthy they are. They recover from the flu in 24 hours, and can eat 5,000 calories of junk every day and never gain an ounce. We're painfully aware that teens can sleep 20 hours on Sunday after staying up all night on Friday and Saturday, and hardly getting any sleep the rest of the week.

We just take their health for granted. We just say… it's youth.

We watch in awe their boundless energy but we don't make the connection between this zest and resilience and hormones. Yes, it is youth, but youth is due in large part to the overabundance of the right hormones in the correct balance. Scientifically speaking, thyroid, growth hormone, estrogen, and testosterone (just to name the top players) rev up the system and stimulate energy production at the cellular level. Teens' metabolic rates are high; they burn fat and they move fast and furious. Muscles are built overnight and the aggressive and optimistic outlook on life makes them feel immortal. Progesterone balances the energizing hormones by softening their impact, moderating the amount of growth and energy produced, and allowing for rest and renewal. This explosion of hormones occurs in the adolescent's body for one reason, and one reason only: to prepare for reproduction.

Don't get me wrong—I don't want to relegate the human species to being only baby-making machines. But that is precisely what hormones do and why our species survives. Our hormones don't care that we are evolved, intelligent humans. They don't care about the latest trends or celebrity sightings. They don't care about popularity or social or personal success. All they care about is that we perpetuate our species. This situation leaves us needing to understand how our hormones work to protect us, how to be clear about when their balance is off and at the helm ready to correct imbalances with treatments that are safe, replenishing the hormones to keep us young and healthy indefinitely. None of us suffers from antidepressant deficiencies. For that matter, no drug makes up for well-balanced hormones in human identical formulations.

Twenties

Moving on to our late teens, early 20s, in better control of our hormones, still not quite mastered, we just enjoy life ruled by them. We have learned to live with our youthful identity, young and wild. Socially, we can tolerate adults just a tad better, although we still doubt their worth. We know we are better and smarter than the older folk but we have acquired some of the tools we need to integrate into society.

What happens next?

We instinctively search for a mate, someone to have children with. Socially, we party, focus on our looks, maybe get an education, find a job, dress cool, work out like crazy to get bodies to compete with the airbrushed celebrities on the covers of magazines. Or maybe we don't follow the crowd. Maybe we leave the rat race and join the Peace Corps, move to a Third World country and take care of those in need or move to a self-sustaining community and live a simpler, energy-efficient life. And while we believe we are following our dreams, instinctively we are searching for the perfect life, the perfect mate, the perfect place to reproduce ourselves.

On the outside social mores define our behavior and looks while on the inside, our hormones protect us from harm and push us ever so gently to perpetuate our species. Heart attacks, cancer and strokes are not common in the 20-year-old age group. You know how the saying goes that the young think they are immortal? Truth be told, they are. Their mission makes them immortal and hormones protect and make sure that goal is achieved no matter how much damage we cause to our bodies with bad habits and bad lifestyles.

The 20s and early 30s is when women tend to get pregnant. When pregnant we are protected from harm: estrogen and progesterone levels are sky-high. We don't get sick, we just glow. We gain weight and yet there are limited and rare problems associated with the weight gain that practically disappear when we give birth. Overall, bones get stronger, hair gets thicker, skin is wrinkle-free, women feel sexy and sleep well (at least until the third trimester) while hormones just do their job.

High estrogen stimulates bone production, protects the heart, keeps our arteries flexible and clear of plaque, stimulates serotonin production, keeping spirits high; life is just great. All at least until the last few weeks of the pregnancy, when most women are ready to be done with it. It is during pregnancies that hormone levels are literally astronomic and it is consistently during this time that most women are healthy and thriving.

This situation begs the question: If estrogen causes cancer, why doesn't the incidence of cancer skyrocket during pregnancy?

This is a time in our lives when we are living a scientific experiment- we are watching how high estrogen levels affect every organ in the body. If we are healthy during pregnancy, it is proof positive that our own estrogen is not a dangerous hormone but rather a safe protector of youth and health, a supporter and enhancer of life, ours and that of the fetus growing inside us.

Even statistically speaking, pregnant women have the lowest incidence of cancer, heart attacks, and strokes when compared to any other group.

IVF/IUI/*Infertility*

The only caveat here are women who have suffered with infertility possibly as a side-effect of long-term use of birth control (made of synthetic/nonhuman identical hormones that suppress our own hormone production), genetic or mechanical factors (e.g., blocked tubes from scarring as a result of old infections), hereditary malformations and other pathologies, who had to undergo IVF treatments (involving versions of synthetic/nonhuman identical hormones). These women may be at higher risks of disease as well as premature ovarian failure after the treatments and may be unable to carry pregnancies to term. The treatments used to impregnate these women sometimes involve strong medications and hormone stimulation with unknown long-term effects. The goal is solely to get the woman pregnant at any cost, not to keep her healthy.

Thirties

Once we found our mate and started a family, we are following the physiologic imperative of our lives and hormonally speaking we are on automatic pilot for the next 15-plus years. While women are busy raising their expanding families Mother Nature wants our species to thrive and survive. This fact translates into fairly constant healthy hormone balance with rare glitches in the system. Our periods are fairly regular, we maintain our weight unless we gorge on junk and drink too much alcohol, sleep well when time allows but have no problem getting up three times in the middle of the night to take care of kids, and still are full of energy the next day. Because it takes our offspring a minimum of 15 years to become at least physically self-sustaining, our hormone balance and the state of our health has to parallel this timeline. Just think about what it takes to get up with a screaming baby in the middle of the night and conduct business as usual three hours later when the day starts for everybody else. Only a healthy and hormonally well-balanced woman can do all that effectively. Scientifically, hormones continue protecting us for the minimum of 15 years we need to raise the children. Culturally, the story is different. Millennials still live at home after college and the future is unclear about when they will be moving out and getting a job. By the time they're finally launched starting their own search for a mate, or beginning a career, they leave behind an empty nest and a hormonally drained 40- to 50-year-old mother.

Oddly, no one talks about what happens to women after they have a baby or two. Women's lives change dramatically and the expectations of them as mothers, wives, members of the workforce (more than 40 percent of women are the primary breadwinner in the U.S. as of 2015 https://www.americanprogress.org/issues/women/reports/2016/12/19/295203/breadwinning-mothers-are-increasingly-the-u-s-norm/) are enormous and mostly unrealistic. Yet, women just do it all. They raise the children, get up in the middle of the night with the babies, do the laundry, bring in the dry cleaning, shop and cook, work full-time, provide emotional support for husband, family and friends—and that is just in a day's work. Their hormones and their acculturation got them here, yet it is high time for change. By the time kids are out of the house women must be able to enjoy the highest quality of life; *they earned it and deserve it.*

Forties/Fifties

How often do you hear about the couple looking forward to shipping the last kid off to college and making plans for early retirement to play golf and then, boom! The wife gets breast cancer. Or, boom! The husband has a heart attack.

Fortunately for most the transition is not so traumatic. Not everyone gets a heart attack or cancer upon retiring. However, lots of changes suddenly occur at this age that must be addressed. There you are, ready to exhale, to reclaim your old romance or maybe even start a new life. Of course, that assumes you are among the lucky few who have not been damaged by the fluctuations in the economy, whose marriage has survived two decades of stress, or someone who can actually afford to retire.

Not so fast. While you're making plans for the next phase of your life you suddenly start sweating in the middle of the night and find that you can no longer deal with the simplest of problems. Overnight, you become a human blimp, your sex drive is gone, and your joints are aching so much you'd rather stay in bed and pull the covers over your head. What is going on here? It's a dirty trick Mother Nature has just played on us. Our job is done, we have accomplished our goal; we reproduced successfully, raised the offspring, and thus secured the propagation of our species.

We are no longer needed so Mother Nature will just get rid of us. We have now become road kill.

Ruthlessly, Mother Nature removes the high octane fuel—our hormones—that protected us from harm and kept us healthy when we were "useful." Once the hormones leave the process of rapid aging accelerates. With advancing age we get sick; blood pressure goes up, we develop heart problems, diabetes, cancer, strokes, arthritis, depression. We become riddled with chronic illnesses, stooped over with thinning brittle bones, endure failing eyesight, lose our sense of smell, hearing, and memory.

So, what is the difference between being young and healthy and old and sick? You know it! It all starts and ends with our hormones. If you are young (and useful, according to Mother Nature), here is your profile. You're brimming with hormones, you're pimply, menstruating, moody, your perspiration has a strong and pungent odor, and you want to have sex—all the time. It might be simplistic, but I tell you, it's a sure way to identify your position on the food chain.

Once you've had kids and they are grown, you are no longer useful and your hormones just leave you. The dwindling hormone levels cause you to get depressed, gain weight (especially that spare tire around your waist) and get bloated, while sleep is nothing short of a nightmare. Sex becomes a chore, your vagina dry like the Sahara, and your skin starts to sag. All the fillers, Botox, lasers, vampire facials, and plastic surgery can't hide the depleted feeling inside your body or make you feel 30 again.

As long as you are young and have the potential to make babies, estrogen, progesterone, testosterone, all hormones will protect you. Ovaries, testes, adrenals, and thyroid will produce the exact quantities of hormones your body needs to stay in optimal health. When you are done having babies, they've grown up and can physically take care of themselves, you are no longer needed. So hormone production just turns off. Your body will betray you and you will get old.

It sounds pretty depressing but it's true, and the clearer you are on the facts, the more likely you can correct the situation.

All of the preceding is just theoretical physiology, and it does not have to apply to any of us if we don't want it to. After all, we put a man on the moon 50 years ago and live in a world where everything you want to know is on Google. We certainly and safely know how to fool Mother Nature and extend our existence by replenishing our hormones and living healthy and productive lives into very advanced age. All we have to do is supplement the waning hormones, change our diet, get moving and keep up the level of exercise, improve our sleep patterns, and put a positive perspective on life and I assure you we can prevent our decline indefinitely. My patients and I have been doing it for more than 25 years.

Why would anyone in their right mind ever question this easy solution?

It goes back to our doctors and the WHI study that said hormones are bad for you. The truth is, it all boils down to the kind of hormones we use. Synthetic/nonhuman identical hormone replacements don't work as well as bioidentical/human identical hormones. Science has proven it repeatedly since the early 1940s. The fact is we never really needed the Women's Health Initiative (WHI) study to find this out. Natural/bioidentical/human identical hormones do work. Just look around and you will notice the growing numbers of both men and women who are defying age, feeling and looking young well into their golden years. You too can, and should, be one of these people.

CHAPTER 3

Symptoms of Hormone Imbalance Occur at All Ages

Chapter 2 taught us that during our reproductive years, we are healthy because the high levels of sex hormones we produce protect us from illness. Of course, that goes along with the fact that we are also young.

Even though most young people are healthy, statistically speaking the system is not perfect. Identifying and understanding the imperfections in our hormone balance that occur during our youth raises self-awareness, helping us protect ourselves from health problems as we age. The more awake we are when we are young, the easier the transitions in our life are.

Hormones do not protect us from *all* harm. Like a computer system, the human body does crash on occasion. The hormone balance gets thrown off even in the healthiest of people at the peak of their youth. When the hormone balance is off, we experience symptoms. Not every young woman will experience symptoms of hormone imbalance, but most women will at different times in their lives. How well we manage our own premenopause, perimenopause, menopause, and postmenopause depends on the understanding of episodes of hormone imbalance that occur at all ages.

Hormone Balance and Symptoms

When our hormones are in balance, our bodies function like well-oiled engines; when the balance is off, we become squeaky wheels. Tiny changes in hormone levels, imperceptible to the most sensitive lab tests, produce significant symptoms. It is the suddenness of these minute changes in hormone levels that give us symptoms at all stages and ages in life.

Our present knowledge and laboratory testing cannot measure these fluctuations. Blood tests offer little help as we desperately try to feel better and doctors don't understand the hormone connection and cannot help us. If no disease label can be placed on the patient, outdated conventional medicine simply has no idea how to treat us.

Since our most up-to-date high-tech tests only provide a snapshot, a moment in time and not what occurs over real time in our body, the only realistic and most reliable diagnostic tool remains, "How do you feel?" To save yourself from harm you must use "How do you feel?" as the gold standard, and connect "How do you feel?" with symptoms and ultimately to hormone imbalances.

Notice how the same symptoms (hot flashes, night sweats, insomnia, weight gain, palpitations, and so forth) you experienced at 20 but ignored because they occurred infrequently and/or your doctor told you they weren't anything serious, become overwhelming at 40, and incapacitating at 60.

It is crucial to realize that symptoms of hormone imbalances occur at all ages throughout our lives. If we recognize the connection between the symptoms and hormone imbalance and treat them with natural/bioidentical/human identical hormones we effectively protect ourselves from diseases of aging. I have been making these connections with more than 20,000 men and women in our practice ranging in ages from teens to 80s for the past 20 years and the results are consistent and reproducible. The results of our work are nothing short of miraculous and leave both our doctors and our patients wondering why everyone else isn't doing the same thing.

Identified by decades, let's look at symptoms of hormone imbalance to help us make them easier to understand and less confusing.

Symptoms of Hormone Imbalance in Your Teens

▶ Acne
▶ Mood swings
▶ Headaches
▶ Menstrual cramps
▶ Occasional sleep disturbances
▶ Occasional weight issues

Acne

Acne is a symptom of hormone imbalance.

Louise was 14 when her mother brought her to see me. She was a late bloomer and had gotten her period that year. Suddenly, her beautiful face was covered with pimples and she had weird headaches, irregular periods, and fatigue before her periods started. The dermatologist wanted to put Louise on birth control pills and Accutane (Accutane is associated with birth defects so every woman who takes it must be on birth control pills according to conventional medical protocol). Her mother opted for working with me because my approach is known to be less aggressive and more individualized.

Turns out Louise was a totally normal teen in need of gentle support while her body matured and adjusted to the effect of hormones and found its natural balance. Acne, headaches, fatigue around the period are all symptoms of hormone imbalances

31

needing a combination of supplements and progesterone (human identical). After checking her blood tests, I placed Louise on 50 mg progesterone in skin cream (Procream, at www.eshealth.com) to be taken in the evening applied to her forearms for the two weeks a month before her period starts, Milk Thistle, an herbal liver cleanser, and vitamin B and fish oil. Within three months Louise's periods became regular, her face cleared of acne, and she no longer suffered with headaches or fatigue before her period. A few months later, her body having decided to create better balance, we no longer needed the hormone support and she stopped taking progesterone and she now only uses the Milk Thistle three times a year.

It's normal for early puberty changes to throw off young women's hormone balance. It is totally normal to see young women in their teens and early 20s with irregular periods. During this adjustment period, the balance of estrogen, progesterone, and testosterone is not perfectly tuned. This imbalance, the highs and lows of rapid changes in hormone levels, sometimes present themselves clinically as acne, headaches, fatigue, mood swings, and bloating. Both estrogen and testosterone make oil glands grow and the progesterone present during and after ovulation closes down the pores and offers a fertile ground for pimple growth. The headaches, fatigue and bloating also occur as direct results of hormone swings.

Mood Swings

Mood swings are caused by hormone imbalance.

A straight A student, Louise was the pride and joy of her parents. Beautiful, bright, and friendly, she seemed to be sailing through the tough teen years with great self-confidence while others were struggling. Now that we had taken care of her acne she was doing really well. Her mother, a longtime patient of mine, often told me how lucky she felt to have a child like Louise. She was a bright and constant example for her younger siblings.

Things went well until Louise turned 17. The change occurred practically overnight. "It was extremely sudden," her mother told me, desperate for advice. One day Louise's personality dramatically changed. What once was a home of happy, open communication turned into door slamming and isolation. A different Louise emerged.

While still a good student, Louise stopped talking to her parents, siblings and most of her friends. She became miserable and intolerant. Her clothes were just like her mood, dark and dreary. She dyed her hair purple and in spite of her parents' threats she started to come home with a new tattoo every few weeks. She spent hours in her room, on the computer, blasting heavy metal music, and rarely came out for dinner. If anyone ever dared ask her what was wrong, Louise attacked. Everything wrong in her life was her parents' fault. Louise's mother took her to a therapist for five sessions. Louise spent the time blankly staring at the wall or at her green-with-black polka dot-painted fingernails.

After many years of being privileged to see teens in action I tell their parents the same thing: "Give them a chance. While things seem strange and impossible now, by the time they turn 20 or 21 and you will be best friends again. You will rapidly move from being a total embarrassment and annoyance to being smart and a worthwhile advisor and most trusted support system. Teens are just trying to separate from you to develop their own identity." To get there it may take almost a decade and lots of difficult days and nights mostly for the parents.

While we each have our own inborn personality, there is no doubt that teens are directly, deeply, and seriously affected by the rapid rise and fall of their sex hormones. The sudden surges followed by precipitous drops in hormones without a doubt propel the most docile teen into a possessed child with the speed of light. A clear-skinned youth will sprout a crop of pimples the day of the prom, or worst of all, a smart young woman will suddenly lose her self-confidence.

Changes in thyroid function affect the teen's moods, acne, sleep issues and weight as well. Sadly, you will seldom hear this from your family doctor or gynecologist. Blood tests won't help. Understanding the impact of hormones and trusting your gut as a parent are the best and safest tools you have.

Stress Changes Hormone Balance

We all know the negative effects prolonged and negative stress have on our bodies. But did you notice that stress makes pimples grow, changes people's personality, and affects sleep and appetite? Of course, you say, but why? Because stress causes immediate and drastic changes in hormone levels.

The best-known physiologic reaction to stress is the "fight and flight" mechanism. Our ancestors who lived in caves and had to protect themselves from attacks by wild animals and other dangers reacted instinctively through their hormones. They did not have the ability to think before they acted. At the core of the mechanism that saved their lives was a simple but most powerful hormone.

Cortisol is the hormone our adrenal glands make to protect us from danger. It is released every time our body or mind thinks we are about to get hurt. To the body, stress means danger. When cortisol is released to help us run away from harm, our immune system is activated. Progesterone and insulin levels drop. This is important because the more time we spend under stress, the more our hormones fall out of balance. The results: increased energy production, accumulation of toxic waste products, faster aging, and ultimately permanent organ damage as manifested in chronic diseases (arthritis, diabetes, heart disease, high blood pressure, and so on).

Symptoms of Hormone Imbalance Occur at All Ages

Our hormones prepare us to fight or run away from the danger we perceive. This mechanism works well in the wild where stress indeed is a matter of life and death. It doesn't work so well in our society where stress may be caused by simple facts like who is more popular in school, how friends treat us, or how we perform on an exam. The cortisol release in response to the perceived "fight and flight" situation, no longer appropriate in our society, creates further hormone imbalances that manifest as acne, fatigue, headaches, weight gain, and mood swings. The teen's body will try to right this hormone imbalance. But the symptoms appear so quickly it may take months or years to get the overall balance pitch perfect.

During this time parents desperately seek help. The help need not come from antidepressants, birth control pills or other medications that affect the entire body and leave short- and long-term undesirable side-effects (infertility, blood clots, memory loss, sleep disturbances, depression, and so on). Teaching children to cope with stress early on in life and flattening those cortisol spikes are the first steps. Understanding the instinctive reaction to stress is based on an old, outdated but highly destructive mechanism and protecting the teen is crucial. Medication is rarely the answer since teens or even adults for that matter are not suffering from "lack of antidepressants" or "need for synthetic hormones to suppress their natural hormone production."

Teaching teens to stop reacting to everything, discouraging drama and setting adult examples of dealing with issues consistently helps raise successful adults. When needed supplementation with natural/bioidentical/human identical hormones is the second step. Natural/bioidentical/human identical hormones are molecularly identical to the teen's own hormones and their action is so gentle, they can easily right the balance and eliminate the symptoms. (The hormones we use in teens are progesterone, thyroid, and adrenal support depending on the individual patient's situation.)

Symptoms of Hormone Imbalance in Your Twenties

▶ Postpartum depression

▶ Night sweats

▶ Infertility

▶ Weight gain

▶ Mood swings

▶ Recurrent urinary tract infections/cystitis

▶ Recurrent vaginitis

Postpartum Depression

In our culture one's 20s is synonymous with "party time." From the physiologic standpoint, beautifully synchronized, our hormones keep us vibrant, healthy, and ready to enjoy life. Many also start to reproduce during this decade, and they start having families. Hormonally, childbirth and its aftermath should go without a hitch yet occasional problems do arise. When they do, we are left baffled and without answers or worse yet, with the wrong answers.

Here's the story of a patient who exemplifies what too many women go through at this stage of life.

Leanne had her first child, a healthy 7-pound, 8-ounce boy, at 24. She and her husband were ecstatic. Leanne went back to work as a school nurse when the baby was 6 weeks old and her mother took care of him during the day. Less than two years later the next baby was born, this time a fair-haired baby girl weighing 7 pounds and perfectly healthy. Leanne and her husband beamed with joy. Their marriage worked, they were blessed with two gorgeous children, and Leanne's mom was still pitching in. Eight weeks after the baby's birth Leanne was supposed to go back to work. However, this time things changed dramatically. She suddenly couldn't get out of bed. At first she thought she was sick and rested a few days. She had chills, sweats, and felt run-down. She didn't even have the strength to see her kids and was thrilled when her mom took them for a few days. Leanne just sat in bed. She didn't go on IG, FB, watch TV, or play games. She didn't even text her friends, which was usually her favorite activity.

A week later, Leanne's husband took her to their local doctor. She had tests done for Lyme disease and a general blood panel. All results came back normal. No one ever thought to check Leanne's hormones since they are not something most doctors are trained to look into or consider in the evaluation of a patient. In fact, Leanne clearly remembered her gynecologist, at her six-week follow-up visit, telling her she was in fine shape and should start having sex and could go back to work. For one second she wondered why the gynecologist never asked her what she wanted to do. But then she forgot about it.

So what was wrong with her? She could barely get out of bed. She asked for a leave of absence from work. The school doctor examined her and also found nothing wrong with her. Both Leanne and her husband were convinced she was losing her mind. So she went to a psychiatrist, who promptly started her on an antidepressant. Leanne slept for three days and nights. When she woke up she got out of bed and came to see me. After blood tests for her hormone levels and listening to her story in detail, it was very clear she had postpartum depression and needed a little progesterone and lots of hugs and kind support from her husband, who by now was afraid to come near her, not understanding what ailed her. He gladly agreed to participate in her treatment.

Leanne got better in one week.

Night Sweats

I had my first baby at 27. I was healthy and had a great pregnancy. I worked until the day I delivered and went back to work two months later.

Oddly, when my baby was less than 2 months old I woke up in the middle of the night drenched in a terrible sweat. At the time, I was practicing conventional medicine and because traditional training is very limited, I thought the only reasons for night sweats could be tuberculosis or severe blood infections. You can only imagine how terrifying the experience was. There I was with a newborn thinking I was deathly ill. Fortunately, by the morning, I was feeling fine and without fever or other signs of major illness, I just moved on with my life.

When I returned to work a few weeks later I remembered the incident and started asking my fellow physicians—mostly men— if they had heard about similar symptoms from patients soon after deliveries. No one had heard of it. I went to the library and researched night sweats in postpartum women in the medical literature and found no mention of the problem. I went back to work and moved on.

As the years passed and I specialized in hormones in wellness and disease prevention, I realized the night sweat episode I experienced was normal and was the result of sudden changes in hormone levels.

Later, when I started teaching doctors about hormones I remembered this episode. Routinely, we started to ask our young women patients about night sweats after having babies. More than 80 percent of those questioned answered yes.

To this day most obstetricians have never heard of postpartum night sweats. Could be the problem comes from the lack of interest in the woman once the baby is born. When questioned, most women feel totally abandoned by their doctors once the baby is born. It's odd how quickly a woman goes from having weekly ultrasounds, blood tests, and visits to the obstetrician while she is pregnant to total abandonment once the baby is born. It's strange because most obstetricians do notice how attached women become to them during the pregnancy. Although we all know pregnancy isn't a disease, our society has medicalized it, which means treating the woman like a sick patient. Once all that care and attention are gone, women suffer from total neglect, although it is totally covert. The doctors' jobs are to make sure the woman delivers a healthy baby. Once the baby is born, it becomes all too apparent the doctor doesn't always represent the woman's best interests.

The medical profession, in fact, only knows how to address problems during pregnancy and offers no tools to help women adjust to their new lives as mothers and wives. "You can have sex again after six weeks" is what most obstetricians tell the woman at the six-week postpartum visit. What about the fact that most women don't feel or look like their old selves yet? Maybe they're not interested in sex after six weeks? What about the fact that most women are exhausted from being up all night with a screaming baby? They are told that is normal and they should go back to their lives. Seems ironic. What defines normal in their new life? This is a very important part of a woman's life and the care she receives must support and encourage her, not minimize her importance.

What Happens Hormonally After Delivery?

The high levels of estrogen and progesterone our healthy bodies make to support the growth and development of the fetus in the womb suddenly drop when the baby is born and they are no longer needed. This sudden drop in hormone levels, the arrival of new hormones on the scene (oxytocin, prolactin), albeit normal, along with the complete life changes a baby brings to the woman may manifest as depression, weight fluctuations, loss of sex drive, and night sweats in many.

Every woman who has a baby experiences a sudden drop in estrogen, progesterone, and HCG levels and a rise in oxytocin and prolactin levels (see Appendix A). When the hormone levels change, symptoms may surface and they often go ignored because women think they are alone and no one else feels them. Nothing could be further from the truth.

The drop in hormone levels after childbirth protects women from far greater harm. Keep in mind hormone levels are high to maintain and support the growth of the fetus in her womb. What would happen if, once the baby was born, levels of estrogen and progesterone just stayed up? That could be lethal. Without the need to support another life, the high hormone levels would literally kill the woman. Too much of hormones would affect negatively all systems: heart, lung, brain, and so forth. Once the baby is born, we must get rid of the high hormone levels as quickly as possible to get back to normal.

However, sometimes in the process of resetting the hormone levels, the body overshoots its goal. Too much of one hormone drops too suddenly, especially in a sensitized, emotionally stressed, or genetically predisposed woman, and that may result in significant symptoms.

The time after a baby is born is known by smart ob/gyns as the "fourth trimester." It's a time in a woman's life where both outside and inside her body many changes happening simultaneously can be overwhelming. If you've just had a baby and are having physical symptoms which you've been told "shouldn't exist," don't ignore them to be nice, or think you are alone. Never allow an uninformed or inconsiderate doctor to reject the validity of your symptoms. I want you to be prepared to listen to *your* body and get the proper help.

Infertility

The area of infertility is a trillion-dollar, constantly expanding business within the field of obstetrics and gynecology. Many causes for infertility have been identified. While some are mechanical, like blocked tubes or undeveloped uterus or ovaries, quite often the cause is hormone imbalance. Examples include:

▸ Inadequate quality or quantity of progesterone produced by the corpus luteum (after ovulation). (See Appendix A.)

▸ Imbalances in levels of estrogen and progesterone negatively impacting implantation and survival of the fertilized ovum into the uterus.

▸ Hormone imbalances preventing fertilization of the egg by the sperm.

▸ Low DHEA levels. (See Appendix A.)

▸ Low testosterone levels.

▸ Antibodies to sperm or fertilized egg.

▸ Low thyroid frequently undiagnosed. (Note: Most gynecologists do not routinely test your thyroid or know how to interpret the results should they even perform them.)

▸ Long-term use of birth control pills has also been correlated to increased incidence of infertility (birth control pills suppress our own hormone production, thus effectively putting its user in a state of chemical menopause).

Hormone problems are often the root cause of infertility in women of all ages.

As women delay having children into their 30s and even 40s, more infertility problems arise, leading to more ethical and physiologic issues surrounding pregnancy, egg freezing, IVF, IUI, embryo donations, and so on. At that time, women make life-changing decisions while focusing entirely on getting pregnant, often without thought for the consequences of these decisions. Some of the consequences, like early menopause, will change the rest of their lives.

Only after the baby is born and many women enter early menopause does the realization of the complicated issues of childbearing with IVF become clearer. Sadly, few make the connection between IVF and early menopause. Steps to correct the problems must be undertaken immediately, or the woman may spend many decades suffering in silence.

Symptoms of Hormone Imbalance in Your Thirties

▶ Bloating
▶ PMS
▶ Migraines
▶ Breast tenderness
▶ Decreasing attention span (scattered thinking)
▶ Weight gain
▶ Irritability

As we move on to our 30s we notice increasing numbers of symptoms showing up. To better understand what happens to our bodies in our 30s, please look up the function of the corpus luteum in Appendix A, and the changes that occur as we get older.

As a quick reminder, the corpus luteum manufactures progesterone to prepare the body for pregnancy. If the woman does not get pregnant, the production of estrogen and progesterone shuts down. The corpus luteum dies and we get our periods.

The same scenario goes on every month for a minimum of 30 years. And all the while the presence of a period makes us think time isn't changing anything else in our bodies. While physically we may look the same between our 20s and 40s, the fact is, hormonally, things are changing.

For the moment, let's look at pure physiology. Both outside and in, a woman in her 30s isn't as youthful as a woman in her 20s. While a few crows' feet may begin to appear and hips may be a little wider, more significant signs of aging are taking place inside the body.

The corpus luteum does not make the same quality or quantity of progesterone as it did in your 20s and that is crucial. The decrease in the quality and quantity of progesterone translates into increasing symptoms in your 30s.

Mary is a normal woman in her 30s. Two children, good job, decent marriage, works a lot, takes care of her family, and is very social. Before her periods she finds herself practically bedridden with headaches. No headache treatment or neurologist has figured a solution yet. The first half of the month, right after her period ends, she feels great and is a veritable Energizer bunny going to the gym 4 to 5 times a week and enjoying her life. After she ovulates (around day 15 of her cycle) she starts to feel bloated, craves salt and sugar, gets tired, no longer goes to the gym, and gets horrible headaches while her sex drive plummets the last week of the cycle.

Mary is generally very happy and her life is proceeding according to plan but would give anything to get rid of the belly bloat, get a little more oomph in her sex life and certainly get rid of those insane headaches.

Although she has seen many doctors, she has found no relief. No one checked her hormones or even connected the problems to hormone imbalances. She was offered antidepressants and birth control pills, painkillers, diuretics, and certainly extensive neurologic work-ups, which invariably found no diagnosable problems. When I saw her, spent a couple of hours going over her story, performed blood tests, and looked at her body composition, I found her thyroid level low. As I listened to the consistency in her story (all the symptoms always occurred the second half of her cycle), I realized she needed a boost with progesterone. Hence, a little supplemental progesterone for the two weeks before her period and a few supplements including vitamin B complex, fish oil, and turmeric (I'll explain why later on). By the next cycle she felt like her old self and even went to a Botox party because, as she said, she felt 20 again and wanted to look it.

Bloating

Bloating is a common symptom that occurs the second half of the cycle, usually after ovulation. It is characterized by swelling in the middle section of the body and in the extremities. Common complaints include a tight feeling of pants or skirts, abdominal discomfort even after a small meal (or just water), tight-fitting rings, dents left on the shins by snug-fitting socks that leave marks on your skin, swollen calves, puffy eyes in the morning, and a ballooning midriff soon after eating most foods.

Water retention in our cells is what causes us to feel the bloat. Holding onto water is often triggered by increased levels of estrogen and poor quality progesterone to balance the estrogen. Elevated levels of estrogen send water into the individual cells; whether they are in your intestines, stomach, or fat cells on your belly, the result is bloating.

Low progesterone from poor quality or no ovulation fails to provide balance and we are stuck with middle-section bloat and the sudden spare tire. Balancing the hormones with progesterone, thyroid, and adrenal support will help tremendously but also changing the diet is critical. An anti- or de-bloating diet involves eliminating milk and milk products (dairy) and attempting to limit carbs, salty foods, and gluten for a while, as well as coffee and alcohol, while adding celery, cucumbers, and other vegetables with diuretic qualities,.

Probiotics are excellent supplements to add in general to improve absorption of nutrients in the gut, improve immune function and support hormone balance.

PMS—PMDD

What's the update on PMS? And what is premenstrual dysphoric disorders (PMDD)? As women enter their 30s, medical labels for symptoms occurring during the menstrual cycles appear. Oddly, when asked, women in their teens and 20s also experience these symptoms but no labels follow them. So why label them in our 30s?

The epidemic of PMS and PMDD oddly enough surfaced in the early 2000s with FDA approval of antidepressants to treat them. When looking deeper into the situation, stress rises to the forefront of the causative factors. Women in their 30s lead more complicated and complex lives—work, relationships, children—while all the while trying to stay young and attractive. I don't believe we are in the throes of an epidemic of psychiatric illness, we are just highly stressed, our lives are very complicated and our bodies respond with symptoms. Sadly, too many antidepressants and other psychotropic drugs are approved by the FDA, are well marketed and make billions of dollars for their manufacturers. This situation alone explains the overabundance of pseudo disease labels and the massive recommendations for treatments with these highly addictive drugs of questionable effectiveness.

The issue of hormone imbalances makes a difficult situation almost unbearable. This time the culprit is primarily progesterone and often thyroid and no antidepressant will make up for the lack of the hormones.

When the quality and/or quantity of circulating progesterone isn't sufficient, estrogen becomes the dominant hormone. Estrogen in overabundance may make you angry, edgy, short-tempered and anxious. At the same time, too much estrogen increases water content of cells in your brain, making thinking fuzzy and unfocused.

The cause of the problems is never lack of antidepressants but rather hormone imbalance (which includes thyroid and adrenal) along with the constantly mounting stressors in our lives.

Breast Tenderness

There is a plethora of causes for breast tenderness and breast cancer should never be at the top of your list. Unfortunately, that isn't the case. A 36-year-old woman came in to see me with a history of terribly sore breasts for almost five years. She had multiple mammograms, ultrasounds, MRIs, and a few biopsies but the results were always negative. With two friends suffering with breast cancer this woman was worried sick. She went to her gynecologist and primary care physician complaining of sore breasts and they kept sending her for tests. The woman was so scared it was heartbreaking. After spending time talking to her, looking at her blood levels, and examining her, I realized the most likely variable in the mix was her IUD (intrauterine device), Mirena, which she had for five years, as long as her symptoms. Mirena is an IUD that contains levonorgestrel, a synthetic progestin, that is released into the bloodstream and sometimes causes breast tenderness and other side-effects. Once the IUD was removed the breast tenderness disappeared within two weeks. Sadly, instead of having the IUD removed as a first step when she complained of sore breasts, the poor woman spent five years having tests and biopsies that could never cure the problem.

I cannot stress the importance of working with a doctor who listens and cares. Only a doctor who is open to the possibility that IUDs, birth control pills, or other medications may cause the problem will protect you by first removing them rather than attacking you with tests and biopsies and telling you drugs or an IUD isn't related to your problems. The longer I practice medicine the more convinced I become the majority of problems are caused by medications, foods, stress, and other lifestyle issues that are easily improved by making honest and correct connections. Then watch the symptoms disappear.

Migraines

Migraines and headaches are the bane of many a woman's existence. Causes are many and often go undetected. Whether it is a mechanical problem stemming from misalignment of the head and neck, musculoskeletal problems, sinus issues, food allergies, medication interaction, poor sleep habits, or strain from exercises, a caring doctor will work with you to narrow the possibilities. And, of course, many headaches are caused by hormone imbalances.

Women with predisposition for migraines often start experiencing severe headaches around the time of menstruation. Headaches may be linked to low progesterone, sensitivity to estrogen, thyroid and adrenal imbalances, and other medications directly affecting hormones.

Often women on birth control pills and other synthetic hormone replacement suffer with migraines, unlike human identical hormones. Birth control pills are made with synthetic/ nonhuman identical estrogens and synthetic progestins. Their direct action is to suppress the normal sex hormone production and obliterate the natural fluctuation of hormones that occurs in a woman's body over the course of the month. Blood hormone levels in women on birth control pills reveal low or no estradiol or progesterone. This is a direct consequence of the effect of birth control pills, which is to suppress the entire hypothalamus-pituitary-adrenal-ovarian axis. *Women on birth control pills have the hormone levels of women in menopause.*

Decreasing Attention Span

How often do you walk into a room and wonder why you're there? How often do you sit in a meeting listening intently to the speaker only to realize that you missed the point of the talk? How often do you start a project and don't finish it? Is this the beginning of Alzheimer's? Are 30-year-olds having "senior moments"?

Decades of clinical experience supported by scientific literature offer simple common-sense answers to those who care to find them. Our lives are crazy busy, we have too much responsibility, ever-increasing stress, and fewer self-care outlets (hair and mani-cures, waxing, and eyelash extensions are not really ways to relax and take care of yourself), and less time to fit in all of life's activ-ities. Plus, decreasing estrogen, progesterone, and thyroid levels no longer protect as they did in our 20s. These factors produce a constellation of symptoms including decreasing attention span. Taking medications, or worrying about aging and the possibility for chronic disability, should not be where your mind takes you. If you are the average, healthy 30-something whose life is just too busy and whose hormones need just a bit of help, make your first priority lifestyle adjustment, then hormone balance. Please don't forget. You aren't missing antidepressants from your system, you are missing the proper hormones in the correct balance.

Weight Gain

Many women in their 30s start to gain weight suddenly, having difficulty maintaining ideal body weight. When asked, they often pinpoint the time they lost the battle of the bulge to the birth of their last child. After the last child is born, many women become unable to lose those extra 20 to 30 pounds.

Bad diet? Lack of exercise? No sleep? Stressful relationships?

Of course, that is all true, but aren't the 20s a time when weight loss isn't really a problem? What has *really* changed?

You guessed it, the biggest changes have occurred in the area of our hormone balance. Those beautifully fine-tuned hormones are now starting to go on the blink. Food cravings are common in our 30s. Women tell me, "I never used to like sweets, now it's all about the dessert menu. I just can't stop myself. I've lost all my willpower."

There is a significant connection among our estrogen/proges-terone levels, thyroid, and insulin. The first time we spoke of insulin was when we addressed stress in teens. We said cortisol, the fight and flight hormone, inhibits insulin production.

For the teen, this was a small problem; as we get older, it becomes a much bigger issue. **Insulin** is a hormone made by the pancreas. The pancreas is a long, thin organ neatly tucked under the left side of our rib cage. It has a lot of roles in food digestion but for our discussion the most important role is to control blood sugar levels through the hormone insulin. When insulin is released into our bloodstream, the blood sugar levels drop. The sugar is pushed into the liver for storage. If too much insulin is released, the blood sugar level drops too low. The sudden drop in blood sugar makes us weak, woozy, shaky on the inside, sweaty on the outside, and craving more sugar (sweets and fruit juices are perfect examples of sugars that stimulate insulin production that causes a rapid drop in blood sugar levels). That means that if we eat a candy bar, cake, candy, pasta, pizza, ice cream, bread, muffins, cookies, desserts—all processed sugar—it is absorbed very quickly into the bloodstream, raising our blood sugar level, causing insulin levels to rise and continuing this vicious cycle. If, instead of eating processed sugar, we eat protein, non-animal fats (avocado, coconut, olive oil, nuts) or fiber and natural unprocessed foods, blood sugar levels rise gradually and insulin levels aren't stimulated to spike rapidly. Constantly fluctuating insulin levels are dangerous to our health. The more our cells are flooded with insulin, the less sensitive they become to it, leading to insulin resistance, a significant step toward diabetes and obesity.

So what does all this have to do with our sex hormones? Insulin release is directly connected to progesterone and estrogen levels. Estrogen stimulates insulin release while progesterone tempers it. Diets low in processed sugar will keep the estrogen/progesterone balance healthy and discourage insulin spikes.

As the quality of progesterone made by the corpus luteum decreases, circulating estrogen is no longer balanced by progesterone, more insulin is released more often, and the craving for sugar becomes more prominent. Did you ever notice around your period how desperately you need to eat frequently or else you feel

weak and shaky? It is because the drop in estrogen and progesterone levels stimulate insulin release, causing the blood sugar
levels to drop rapidly. Unfortunately, this domino effect leads to
wear and tear of all body organs and thus aging.

It is a fact that women tolerate low sugar levels better than
men. While men need sugar levels around 90, women are perfectly
normal with blood sugar levels between 50 to 60. When the
hormone balance is off, insulin levels spike out of control. This
situation causes sugar levels to plummet even lower and women
become quickly hypoglycemic; they feel weak, dizzy, shaky, and
sweaty and above all, crave sugars. The older the woman, the less
finely tuned her hormone balance, the more insulin resistance and
sugar cravings, the more symptoms appear and the more rapidly
the aging process progresses. The best way to treat the problem is
to eat protein and non-animal fat every 3 to 4 hours and to avoid
processed sugars at all costs.

Symptoms of Hormone Imbalance and the Appearance of Diseases in Your Forties and Beyond

- Insomnia
- Loss of sex drive
- Hot flashes
- Palpitations
- Night Sweats
- Heart Disease
- Hair Loss
- Digestive Problems (heartburn, GERD, gallstones)
- Weight Gain
- Bone Loss
- Depression

- ► Irritability
- ► High cholesterol
- ► Mood swings
- ► High blood pressure
- ► Bloating
- ► Alzheimer's Disease

By now, it should be obvious that symptoms associated with premenopause, perimenopause, and menopause occur throughout life. Only at menopause, when they increase in frequency and occur all at once, do we become overwhelmed and scared by their destructive effects. If you look back over the previous twenty pages you notice that almost every symptom under the 40-plus heading has appeared before in this chapter. It should be reassuring to see that this is not a sudden development. We experience all these horrible symptoms at other times in our lives. So why allow them to demolish us physically and emotionally at menopause?

Suffice it to say, if we live long enough we will go into menopause and even if we sail through better than the average woman, the symptoms are still there and the long-term damage will catch up with us. So let's identify the problems and solve them just in case you decide you want to feel better.

Hot Flashes

It never ceases to amaze me that women come to see me to help rid them of hot flashes years after they started suffering with them. Women experience hot flashes during their 20s and 30s as well so why don't they seek help then? Most likely, it was because no one raised our awareness to the fact that hot flashes are not just an embarrassing moment in the middle of a board meeting. Their frequency increases at perimenopause and menopause and that's when we begin to notice them. Although there are no scientific studies nor serious monies spent to analyze the origin or significance of hot flashes, from my experience and research they seem to represent a combination of possibilities of which the most likely is the release of pulses of luteinizing hormone by the pituitary gland requesting the ovaries make more estrogen. In most women I treat, hot flashes subside when given estrogen and/or thyroid hormones. The temperature control mechanisms ruled by the hypothalamus and thyroid also get out of balance and contribute to hot flashes.

Auras—premonitions—of hot flashes are common. Most women report they know a hot flash is coming before it actually starts. Awakening from deep sleep by the aura is not unusual and then finding yourself drenched in what is known as a night sweat is the nocturnal version of the hot flash.

The hot flash may last seconds to minutes and feel like your head has been stuck in a furnace, heat crawls up your spine into your hair, your neck is on fire, or your entire body is burning, leading to drenching sweats and cold chills when it's over. Sweating between the breasts is very common.

Everyone agrees, hot flashes are horrible and we'd do anything to get rid of them. While the science behind the causative agents for hot flashes is sparse in research, significant data support the connection between the frequency of hot flashes and the risk of heart disease. Women who have lots of hot flashes may be at higher risk of heart disease. Studies from universities in Israel and other academic institutions seem to support this important connection. The best and only physiologic way to get rid of hot flashes is to take hormones. Estradiol, the natural/bioidentical hormone our bodies make when we are young, is the most effective treatment.

Depression

Estrogen stimulates the production and release of serotonin, the feel-good hormone in the brain. At perimenopause and menopause, estrogen levels drop and serotonin follows. On the outside, the aging process robs us of youthful looks leaving us wrinkled, sallow, and crape-skinned with cellulite and age spots while on the inside we are starting to feel we are falling apart. Joints and back aches, foggy thinking, weight gain, loss of sex drive, depression, you name it. It's all part and parcel of the entire hormone depletion package. Along with the drops in estrogen and serotonin, the decreasing quality and quantity of progesterone, the dropping thyroid, adrenal, and growth hormone levels and the changes on the outside, depression rears its ugly head as age just keeps moving on.

Loss of Sex Drive

Human sexuality is a complex matter. The scientific debate over the seat of sexuality has been raging for many decades. Is sexuality strictly confined to our physical plant, is it all mental or could it be a combination of mind and body? Answers abound but often we may not want to hear them. Take, for instance, the prairie vole, a small, well-studied mammal that takes one partner for life. They nest, have babies, and groom each other (a mammal sign of intimacy). However, once in a while they stray and have sex with other prairie voles. It doesn't change their monogamous behavior beyond the mere act of sex; the vole partners continue living together and sharing all household responsibilities for life. This example raises the question of whether sex is necessarily part of a monogamous relationship; certainly not for the prairie voles.

When it comes to us humans the answer is a bit more complicated. While we are taught monogamy defines a good relationship, and a long relationship is desirable and considered a sign of stability and respected in our culture, all we have to do is look at our celebrities and politicians, next-door neighbors, or even ourselves to realize that sex may be the fly in the ointment of our definition of good and lasting relationships, affecting our perception of them dramatically and constantly. At the end of the day, the decision of how important sex is in our relationships and how we define monogamy is up to each individual or couple.

Getting back to our hormones. When it comes to sex, the connection between mind and body is of utmost importance. Sexuality rarely occurs independent of the mind and hormones make that connection for us. When thyroid, estrogen, progesterone, and testosterone levels are high, sexuality is at its peak (but we are also young and fertile and relationships are new and exciting). When the levels start declining in your 40s, 50s, and beyond, women and men complain of decreasing libido, loss of sex drive, erectile dysfunction, and vaginal dryness. But lest we forget, relationships are by then also decades old.

Vaginal dryness comments such as "feels like sandpaper or the Sahara" don't make sex much of a turn-on. Painful intercourse, diminishing ability to reach orgasm, and recurrent urinary tract infections create a vicious cycle, culminating with decreased frequency of sexual activity and finally no sex at all for many women. As for men, with aging and lack of excitement and passion, erections are less strong or lasting, making sexual intercourse difficult and disappointing for both genders.

But the reality is that sexual intercourse at any age positively impacts many aspects of our life for multiple reasons:

▶ Improves vaginal lining
▶ Increases vaginal secretions
▶ Improves orgasm frequency and quality
▶ Improves a woman's self-image and confidence
▶ Improves mood and outlook
▶ Improves relationships and promotes intimacy

To protect women's sexuality and maintain it there are options we must consider.

Hormone supplementation with bioidentical hormones like estradiol, testosterone transdermal or occasionally low-dose testosterone pellets inserted under the skin, and estriol/DHEA in vaginal tablets and suppositories and vaginal rings will help relieve vaginal dryness, improve vaginal wall thickness and lubrication, and prevent recurrent vaginal and urinary tract infections and vaginal atrophy.

Intimate (communicating, hugging, kissing, caressing, hugging, petting, making out), sexually active relationships, solid self-esteem, confidence, and an optimistic outlook on life guarantee success and a long and rewarding sex life. Old, stale relationships where sex is a chore and intimacy is lacking contribute to further loss of sex drive and self-esteem, which may translate into sexual escapades to improve self-esteem, stroke injured egos, feel desired and youthful, or withdrawal into depression and aging.

Chronic Diseases of Aging

Diabetes, osteoporosis, hypertension, heart disease, cancer, Alzheimer's, and arthritis are common diseases of aging. They occur as the result of many factors: wear and tear, bad eating habits, poor sleep, sedentary lifestyles, processed food, too much alcohol and stress, and genetics, but also because our hormones disappear, removing the mechanism for rebalancing and protecting our health.

Chronic diseases of aging occur in the aftermath of years of chronic inflammation, insults to the system toxic from foods, the environment, and stress. Hormonally, our ovaries stop making estrogen and progesterone, leaving us unprotected from the ravages of age. The same happens with thyroid, adrenals, insulin, serotonin, and growth hormones. With aging, telomeres—the nubs at the ends of our chromosomes that predict longevity—start to shrink. The shorter the telomeres, the shorter the lifespan. This domino effect of changes translates into illnesses, infirmity, frailty, and finally death. However, if we preempt the damage caused by the permanent loss of hormones, supplement thyroid, adrenal, and even growth hormones, forestall telomeres from shrinking, significantly improve our diets, continue and expand our physical activities, maintain muscle mass, sleep 7 to 8 hours a night, take specific supplements, and delete stressful, negative relationships from our lives, we can prevent illnesses and be productive and enjoy life until our last day. It's a lot easier than you think; it's all in the realm of your reality.

Osteoporosis

Estrogen stimulates bone production and inhibits the action of osteoclasts, the cells that break down bone. When the levels of estrogen diminish, this positive effect on the structure of our bones dwindles. Genetic predisposition for osteoporosis, anti-estrogenic medications (tamoxifen, raloxifene, and so on), extended steroid usage (prednisone, medrol, cortef, cortisone, cortisol, and so forth) for various medical problems, eating a diet low in calcium and not supplementing vitamin D, boron, vitamin K, selenium, and zinc, being sedentary, avoiding sun exposure, and extensive use of sunblock—all are contributing factors to osteoporosis. Genetic predisposition and increasing age increase the risk of osteoporosis while hormone supplementation, healthy natural diets, and serious weight-bearing exercises help counteract the problem by slowing its progression. Medication (Actonel, Boniva, Fosamax) is dangerous and has never been scientifically proven to help prevent osteoporosis or truly stabilize and improve bone density without significant side-effects. The aftermath of these drugs is brittle bones that break like glass, leaving us further handicapped and aging even faster. The solution is *never* in a drug. It's in your lifestyle.

Heart Disease

By the age of 50, women catch up with men in the incidence of heart disease. Estrogen depletion is the main reason why. Genetics, smoking, obesity, lack of exercise, poor quality sleep, and diets high in animal fat and processed sugars are contributing factors. Unfortunately, until twenty years ago, no study was conducted to evaluate the effects of estrogen deficiency on the female heart and to establish a safe and successful program for prevention of heart disease in women. The PEPI trials, published in *The Journal of the American Medical Association* in 1999 and the *Archives of Medicine* were the first to look at the "Post-Menopausal Estrogen/ Progestin Interventions." Women who had been taking synthetic estrogen (conjugated equine estrogen—Premarin) replacement therapy had a lower risk of getting heart disease after many years of therapy. For those women who took HRT for only a year, the risk of heart disease was the same as for women who did not take HRT at all. Other studies in Europe and the U.S. have shown that using hormones early will improve outcome and prevent heart disease especially when bioidentical/estradiol hormones are used. (See the Danish Study, E3N study in References.)

But the scientific story of hormones took a horribly wrong turn in 1993 to 1994 when the NIH decided to conduct the Women's Health Initiative.

The Women's Health Initiative—A Final Look

The Women's Health Initiative (WHI), that confusing and disastrous study, was developed and conducted under the auspices of the National Institutes of Health (NIH), academic institutions and the generous financial support of Wyeth pharmaceuticals, owner of the Premarin patent and manufacturer of the drug used in the study. The drug, made from pregnant horses' urine, was the only type of estrogen used in the WHI study. Please note, at the time there were other types of hormone preparations that should have been included in the study but were omitted, raising questions about the true intentions of the study (promotion of Premarin and exclusion of its bioidentical counterpart, estradiol). As I explained in Chapter 1, the study, which was supposed to take 8½ years, was stopped abruptly after 5 years in 2002 because women taking Premarin, Prempro, and Provera (nonhuman identical hormones) had a higher incidence of heart attacks, strokes, and cancer than the women who took a placebo. The problems with the study led to 10 years of lost opportunity for women to take natural/bioidentical/human identical hormones which are safe and protect from heart disease and in clinical use for decades before the WHI study.

What was wrong with the study besides the fact that the U.S. government and the academic institutions took money from a drug company to conduct a flawed study aimed at promoting a $2 billion-a-year drug (Premarin)? Well, there were a few other problems:

▶ The study was biased because it excluded natural/bioidentical/human hormones. I've always wondered why the academic institutions didn't insist that more than one type of estrogen and progestin be studied, given that legitimate organizations such as the International Menopause Society clearly stated "all hormones do not behave the same," thus Premarin could not be representative of all estrogen preparations. Clearly, the main reasons were financial. Academic institutions are heavily financed by drug companies so their scope is limited by their sponsors. That is sad because the only scope should be the health of the population it studies and serves.

▶ The women in the study were older, at least 10 years after menopause and the medical community at the time wasn't clear the best time to start hormone therapy for optimal results was as early as symptoms started, most often before menopause.

▶ The women in the study had preexisting conditions (smokers, heart disease, strokes, obesity, arthritis, and diabetes, for example), which made it difficult to tell which of the problems were caused by the hormones studied and which were just aggravated by them or by the passage of time.

▶ The women took the synthetic/pregnant mares' urine hormones (Premarin) orally (by mouth) and many studies before and after the WHI demonstrated that creams, gels, patches, or transdermal (through the skin) formulations of estrogen, may be safer and better absorbed because they aren't metabolized through the liver at the same rate as oral formulations. Estrogen and progestin (Premarin, Prempro, and Provera), especially synthetic/nonhuman identical, is toxic to the liver and alters bleeding parameters, causing higher incidence of blood clots. (All you have to do is look at the insert on your birth control pill. It is synthetic/nonhuman identical estrogen and progestin and it increases the risk of blood clots.)

▶ The results of the WHI do not apply to any other kind of estrogen or progesterone besides Premarin, Prempro, and Provera. There is no such thing as "class effect" (meaning all estrogens and all progesterones behave the same); every type of estrogen and progestogen acts differently, thus the action/effect of one cannot be applied to another.

The Women's Health Initiative was a disaster for women and their doctors in the U.S. and abroad.

In its wake, due to the government involvement and fear of exposure that the funding for the study came from special interest and omitted bioidentical/human identical hormones, the academic centers where the study was conducted together with the NIH made the decision to disseminate to the public and the prescribing doctors the inaccurate fact that "all hormones are dangerous and may cause cancer, heart attacks, and strokes," although no scientific basis for this statement existed then or now.

The FDA requires a black box warning on all FDA-approved hormone preparations including 17-beta estradiol and micronized progesterone, which are bioidentical/human identical and natural. Gynecologists to this day will often tell you that Premarin and bioidentical hormones are the same even though solid scientific data has proven consistently that all estrogens and progestins do not behave the same in the human body.

Bioidentical/human identical/natural hormones are pharmaceutical products manufactured specifically to mimic the hormones our bodies make in real life and they do not act like the hormones made out of pregnant horses' urine studied in the WHI.

Today, millions of women are still suffering with horrible symptoms of menopause because they have been instilled with fear that hormones will cause breast cancer. This is a horrific situation and honestly there is little relief in sight. Scientifically and clinically, as well as statistically, nothing can be further from the truth.

The truth is that while it is sad that 35,000 women die of breast cancer and many of them from complications of its treatment every year, it is also horrific that 350,000 women die of heart disease, which is preventable with the use of the proper hormone supplementation, diet, exercise, sleep, stress management, and honest support from a medical profession whose sole purpose should be to serve the patient's best interest. There are more than 55 million menopausal women in the U.S. today and if treated correctly with bioidentical hormones, changes in diet, exercise, lifestyle, supplements, and stress management without fear or intimidation, they have decades of healthy, contributory lives to look forward to.

Alzheimer's

Lack of estrogen has been directly implicated in the increased incidence of Alzheimer's found in older women. Estrogen's direct effect on the brain is stimulatory while progesterone's effect is balancing and calming. Without the proper balance between estrogen and progesterone, deterioration of the brain can lead to Alzheimer's. Genetics, lifestyle issues, and the poor Western diet are important contributors as well. Multiple studies have raised questions and brought proof about the positive role of estrogen supplementation in the prevention and even slowing of Alzheimer's. Designer estrogens, such as raloxifene, were developed to specifically address the beneficial effects of estrogen on the brain. To date studies have failed to substantiate any of the claims made by these drugs but have substantiated the positive role of real estrogen in the form of estradiol, which is the bioidentical/human identical/natural estrogen.

New studies have also shown that natural/human identical/bioidentical progesterone when used in large doses during acute brain trauma improves outcome better and safer than any FDA-approved drug on the market.

Cancer

The aging process is associated with increasing incidence of chronic and often severe illnesses. Older women and men with low to nonexistent hormone levels have higher incidences of various forms of cancer and heart disease. Before we continue following the unproven tale that hormones cause cancer, let us remember that pregnant women with very high levels of circulating hormones (estrogen, progesterone, testosterone) rarely get cancer. In fact, hormones appear to provide protection from serious illnesses. The connection between cancer and hormones is under constant scrutiny by the global medical community. Since the massive confusion created by the WHI, the rise in cancer risk for women taking synthetic/nonhuman identical hormone replacements (Premarin, birth control pills, and others) has become the source of heated debates.

In Chapter 9, we address the issue of cancer and its connection to synthetic/nonhuman identical and bioidentical hormones based on a thorough and in-depth review of the scientific literature available to date. Unfortunately, many unscrupulous people use the fear cancer elicits to force women into wrong choices in their health care (avoidance of hormones) that lead to poor quality of life and a neverending lineup of tests and procedures without any evidence of improved outcomes or prevention.

As we come to the close of this chapter we have established three crucial facts:

1. Hormones are life-sustaining and the correct type of hormones will protect us.
2. Hormone imbalances cause specific symptoms at all ages and when these symptoms are present they can be easily identified and treated safely with bioidentical hormone formulations.
3. Symptoms of hormone imbalance occur at all ages and are not limited to menopause.

We now also clearly understand what happened to cause so many doctors and women to be afraid of hormones and the facts behind that situation.

In the next two chapters, we will address options for treatments. I will give you a solid overview of the options and prepare you for physicians who may not be as knowledgeable or understanding of your needs. In the end, you will become confident and ready to address your life and hormone balance from the perspective of "true prevention."

CHAPTER 4

Treatment Options
and Conventional Therapies

It is critical for you to know your options. My evaluation of these treatments is based on more than 30 years of clinical experience and solid cutting-edge scientific information. Beyond my personal extensive clinical experience, my staff and I have conducted a thorough and exhaustive research of the literature, both lay and professional. I am invited to speak at conferences in the U.S. and abroad, helping doctors and the public sort out available choices and make smart decisions they can feel confident with.

A day does not go by that I don't hear women agonizing over treatment options either for menopause or symptoms of hormone imbalance in general. Conversations with new patients invariably sound like this:

"Doctor, I have done lots of research, gone online, read magazines and books on the topic of hormone replacement and menopause, and I am lost. Most doctors offer either what is considered conventional, synthetic/nonhuman identical hormone replacement therapy (Premarin or birth control pills), or I go to my acupuncturist, naturopath, chiropractor, or local health food store and take herbal remedies. When I ask about bioidenticals invariably I'm told all hormones are

the same or bioidenticals are snake oil. They also tell me only quacks prescribe them, and they just turn up their noses at me and I feel foolish and get scared. I must admit to having tried practically everything and nothing has really worked to help me feel like my old self again. I am here because I am at the end of my rope. Can you help me?"

Yes, I can.

Working with natural/bioidentical/human identical hormones has been like finding the golden fleece—the safe universal cure for symptoms of hormone imbalance. Before we delve deeper into bioidenticals I want to address some of the other options you will hear and read about. The reason you need to be familiar with alternative and conventional options is simple. Armed with accurate information you can be confident that when you make your decision, it is right for you and you can stand by your decision without doubting yourself or allowing the outside world to intimidate and frighten you.

Conventional doctors, friends, family members, media, the internet, and holistic specialists are there to give advice. Keep in mind all advice is biased. And that includes mine. Pay attention from whence the information comes, educational background, and professional perspective. No one can give you a complete overview of the different treatment options in a 30-minute session or over a cup of coffee. And even if they could, their own bias will come right through, so you must be philosophically aligned if you want to obtain excellent results.

Following is a comprehensive overview of information on the most commonly used conventional and alternative options you will find for the treatment of symptoms of hormone imbalance. Learn about them and then find the right practitioner to work with who will represent your best interest and is able and willing to work with you and change your treatment as you change.

If you feel consistently better, stay with the program you have chosen; if you are dissatisfied or even unsure with the results, move on to other options. Do not feel obligated to stay with one type

The Side-Effect Dilemma

The use of prescription or over-the-counter medications to treat medical conditions invariably creates a high potential for undesirable effects of the drug. Let me explain: A great example is the usual nonsteroidal anti-inflammatory drugs wallpapering the drugstore shelves with all different names for the same product: Advil, Motrin, Aleve, ibuprofen.... They're *exactly* the same drug with differing dosages and the same effect: to decrease pain in your head, joints, muscles, menstrual cramps, you name it. People take them like candy. All their labels warn us they can cause stomach irritation, bleeding, and ulcers. Everybody just ignores the label. Unfortunately, I can't tell you how many problems caused by these drugs. Yet, we keep taking them and covering up for their side-effects with more drugs. How many of you have taken these drugs and then treated the heartburn they caused with Zantac, Pepcid, Tagamet, or Maalox?

That's just the start. The medications you take to treat the side-effects have side-effects as well, and so it goes.

Eventually you realize that you cannot target a single symptom with medication. It's actually a very crazy thing drug manufacturers and doctors would have us believe; one drug, one effect. Where? In a human being? It's plain crazy. No matter what medication you take, whether prescription or over-the-counter, it will always affect your entire body. It's like dropping a pebble into a lake; the ripple effect is far-reaching and cannot be ignored.

of therapy. Some women are afraid to change therapies. Women make treatment choices based on TV ads, the internet, and information from magazines. Conventional choices come from multiple physicians' offices who all too often don't communicate with one another. *No matter what path you follow, the best measurement of how your treatment works is how you feel.* I often see women who have been taking a particular type of hormone or other medication for years not feeling better. They are afraid to tell their doctors. I feel for these women. They are forgetting they are not there to please their doctors. The goal is to take care of yourself. The real success stories come from people who make sure the therapies they follow fit into their lives. There is a time and place for many therapies but the true key to success is to figure out how to combine them, when to take them and for how long. You should feel free and empowered to try every option to find what works for you.

A word of caution before we enter the details of conventional therapies; we humans are works in progress. We are constantly changing, our bodies, our minds, our tastes. If a remedy works today, it may not work tomorrow. You should not be wedded to one treatment. Learn to read the signs your body sends and listen to them. Your body will never lead you astray, but ignoring its signals will. And never forget, as long as we are alive, we change. Our bodies change all the time so don't think that one treatment will be the same forever.

Conventional Methods of Treatment for Symptoms of Hormone Imbalance

Broken down by individual symptoms, here is a simple yet functional list of conventional treatment options.

Fatigue

The most common symptom physicians in clinical practice encounter is fatigue. Long before the patient is diagnosed with a disease, the complaint of fatigue is there for months, if not years.

Fatigue may be caused by multiple reasons:

1. Lack of sleep—length and quality, shift work
2. Bad eating habits
3. Poor sleep hygiene
4. Late exercise
5. Drinking alcohol or caffeinated drinks before bedtime

6. Stress
7. Interruptions from environmental factors (snoring partner, children and pets, other noises)
8. Hormonal issues—low estrogen, low thyroid, low progesterone, and so forth. At perimenopause and menopause, most women become fatigued without being able to identify the cause.
9. Hyperalert states caused by internal stressors, medical problems, or medications.

The overall problem with fatigue is that it is a warning sign that, if left untreated and unattended, becomes a disease.

In conventional medicine, we only look at a few causes of fatigue (anemia, low thyroid, infectious disease, cancer, heart disease) and instead of integrating the patient's life in the discovery process we just wait for disease to declare itself.

Oftentimes in conventional thinking fatigue is misinterpreted as depression and antidepressants are prescribed as well as mood elevators like amphetamines (Adderall or Vyvanse). Over time, dependency occurs while fatigue continues to worsen because its root cause isn't addressed with the medication.

Acne

While topical medications are recommended as first-line treatment for teen to middle age acne, antibiotics like doxycycline are greatly overused.

A young woman of 24 I saw was taking the antibiotic doxycycline for 10 years without interruption, and no physician recommended she stop. The acne persisted until I balanced her hormones and put her on topical creams for her face. Antibiotics have side-effects and over time they destroy your gut flora and create superbugs resistant to the original antibiotic. Yet, doctors prescribe them and patients take them without questioning the end point.

Commonly used prescription and over-the-counter creams, ointments, and washes include BenzaClin, Benzamycin, Cleocin T, Differin, Retin-A, and benzoyl peroxide. The next step for dermatologists and some internists is Accutane. By law, physicians have to follow rigid guidelines when prescribing Accutane. Because it causes severe damage to fetuses, women of childbearing age are not allowed to take Accutane without simultaneously taking birth control pills. The course of treatment is quite long and liver function must be checked through blood tests at short intervals. Another potentially dangerous side-effect of Accutane is depression.

There are many types of laser and dermabrasion treatments available for acne. Because they are not invasive and you don't have to worry about your unborn children or adding another stressor to your life, ask your dermatologist about these options first. And make sure your hormones are well-balanced before undergoing these treatments.

Bloating

Diuretics is the category of medications most frequently used to treat bloating, also identified as water retention, and are available by prescription only. Examples of the most commonly prescribed diuretics are furosemide (Lasix), Maxzide, hydrochlorthiazide, and spironolactone (Aldactone).

As with all medications, they should be used with caution, because their actions extend beyond their diuretic function.

Diuretics deplete your body of potassium (with the exception of spironolactone), make you feel tired, and raise uric acid levels, often increasing the risk for acute gout attacks in older individuals. Take them with a potassium supplement or a banana and do not use them more than a week at a time just for bloating. Sometimes they may mask other issues, and dependency on them is not desirable but quite frequent. Your body may also get used to them and their desired effects no longer achieved. In our practice, we only use spironolactone (Aldactone), a potassium-sparing diuretic with hormone-supporting effects as needed for short periods of time, with good results.

Marilyn travels a lot and is a 43-year-old patient in our practice. Her hormones are easily balanced. She's been working with us for a decade and while she started with irritability, mood swings, weight gain, and night sweats 10 years ago, she is now free of symptoms, has lost more than 20 pounds (and kept them off), and feels great most of the time. The only problem she still occasionally has that hormones and lifestyle changes haven't been able to resolve is water retention, especially on the long trans-Atlantic trips she takes all too often for work. So a regimen of Aldactone 100 mg—two tabs a day for three days after one of her trips—has been doing the trick, and she doesn't need anything else.

Postpartum Depression, Depression, and Mood Swings

Whether you are 15 with mood swings, 20-something with postpartum depression, or 50 in the middle of a major depressive episode, the devastating effects of mood disorders cannot be overstated.

Too often I see women with successful careers, great parents, and involved spouses, who without clear warning become overwhelmed by their life and suddenly incapacitated by depression.

These women are most likely to enter the medical system seeking help through their primary care physicians or gynecologists.

Sadly, the knee-jerk reaction for these doctors is to start these women on antidepressants, and/or send them to a psychopharmacologist.

If you choose the antidepressant medication route, find a good therapist as well. Medication alone will never solve the underlying problems causing your depression. Talk therapy is an absolute requirement. The therapist must work together with the psychopharmacologist to help you get the most out of the medication. Use their expert help only to help choose the most likely medication to improve your symptoms. And do not use medication indefinitely; most situations change and so do your needs. I cannot tell you how many women I see who have been on antidepressants for decades and they cannot identify one single symptom the medication has helped. And the reason they stay on the medications is because these drugs are so addictive you cannot get off them without going into serious withdrawal.

Antidepressants most often used to treat women with depressive episodes are prescription medications that work directly on the brain. The most popular ones increase circulating levels of a hormone called serotonin by blocking an enzyme that metabolizes the serotonin in the brain (SSRIs).

Scientific data has established that people with high levels of serotonin in the brain are in a better mood than those with low levels. Although no one knows exactly why this is the case, a whole series of antidepressants have been developed by the pharmaceutical companies to raise serotonin levels or stop its breakdown. How these drugs really work, no one knows including their manufacturers, the FDA that approved their usage, or the doctors who write the prescriptions.

Over the past 10 years, antidepressants have become the highest selling drugs in the U.S. and a staple in the field of psychiatry, where they have become as popular as vitamins. Prozac, the first blockbuster antidepressant, was referred to as vitamin P in its heyday, the late 1990s and early 2000s. In an attempt to treat the dominant symptoms of mood disorders—depression and anxiety—a wealth of drugs has flooded the market. Pharmaceutical representatives visit the physicians' offices almost monthly with a new cure-all antidepressant or antianxiety drug *du jour*.

If you don't know about antidepressants you probably don't watch TV and are among the fortunate few who don't use them.

For those who take them, it is important to know they all have dangerous side-effects including worsening depression, weight gain, loss of libido, suicidal ideation, stomach problems, emotional disconnect, and many others. Unfortunately, antidepressants are dispensed with impunity by primary care doctors and psycho-pharmacologists at the first complaint of difficulty coping or just thinking we are depressed.

Antidepressants include:

- ▶ **Venlafaxine** (Effexor XR). Venlafaxine may work for some people when other antidepressants haven't. It can cause side-effects similar to those caused by SSRIs. Venlafaxine can raise blood pressure, and overdose can be dangerous or fatal.

- ▶ **Desvenlafaxine** (Pristiq). Desvenlafaxine is similar to venlafaxine and causes similar side-effects. Studies haven't proven any advantage to desvenlafaxine over venlafaxine, and since venlafaxine is available in a generic form, it's generally a more affordable option should anyone seriously consider taking it.

- ▶ **Duloxetine** (Cymbalta). Duloxetine may help relieve physical pain in addition to depression, but it isn't clear yet whether it works better than other antidepressants for pain relief. Duloxetine can cause a number of side-effects. Nausea, dry mouth, and constipation are particularly common. You shouldn't take duloxetine if you're a heavy drinker or you have certain liver or kidney problems.

Atypical antidepressants are medications that are called "atypical" because they don't fit neatly into other categories. Generally, atypical antidepressants cause fewer sexual side-effects than other antidepressants do.

Atypical antidepressants include:

▶ **Bupropion** (Wellbutrin, Wellbutrin SR, Wellbutrin XL). Bupropion has few sexual side-effects. It may also suppress appetite, and it is used to help you stop smoking. People with seizure disorders or who have bulimia or anorexia shouldn't take bupropion.

▶ **Trazodone** (Oleptro). This mild antidepressant is often prescribed as a sleep aid because it can be very sedating. It has been around for many decades and was used for psychotic patients before the newer anti-psychotic medications came to market.

▶ **Mirtazapine** (Remeron, Remeron SolTab). Like trazodone, mirtazapine can be sedating. It may increase lipid levels and cholesterol and it causes mental cloudiness and emotional disconnect.

▶ **Nefazodone.** This antidepressant is also questionably effective, but isn't commonly prescribed because it has been linked to dangerous liver problems.

Tricyclic and tetracyclic antidepressants is a group of older antidepressants that happen to be more effective, but are usually not a first-choice treatment for depression because of numerous side-effects such as dry mouth, constipation, difficulty urinating, sedation, weight gain, and sexual side-effects. Since they are old, they are off-patent, meaning no money can be made off them by their original manufacturer, thus no money is spent marketing them. In some cases, a low dose of a tricyclic antidepressant is added to another antidepressant, such as an SSRI, to increase the antidepressant's effect, which often makes me wonder why use the SSRI altogether if it isn't working well enough and necessitates the addition of another drug. I still recall the many patients with cardiac arrhythmias caused by overdoses of tricyclic antidepressants I saw during my training in the ER at Kings County Hospital.

Tricyclic and tetracyclic antidepressants include: **amitriptyline**, **clomipramine** (Anafranil), **doxepin** (Silenor, Zonalon), **Imipramine** (Tofranil, Tofranil-PM), **trimipramine** (Surmontil), **desipramine** (Norpramin), **nortriptyline** (Pamelor, Aventyl), **protriptyline** (Vivactil), **amoxapine**, and **Maprotiline**.

Monoamine oxidase inhibitors (MAOIs) are used as a last resort because of numerous and potentially dangerous serious side-effects. However, MAOIs can be effective for some forms of depression when other medications haven't worked. Side-effects can include dizziness, dry mouth, upset stomach, difficulty urinating, muscle twitching, sexual side-effects, drowsiness, and sleep problems. MAOIs can cause potentially fatal high blood pressure when combined with certain foods (cheese) and beverages (red wine) and certain other medications.

MAOIs include: **isocarboxazid** (Marplan), **phenelzine** (Nardil), **tranylcypromine** (Parnate) and **selegiline** (Emsam, Eldepryl, Zelapar).

For patients with anxiety and panic attacks also looking for sleep aid at the same time, **Valium**, **Xanax**, **Trazodone**, **Klonopin**, and **Ativan** are most commonly prescribed.

Before you enter the world of antidepressant medication, you might find it interesting to learn that multiple articles over the span of two decades, in many medical journals including the *American Journal of Psychiatry* and in *Obstetrics and Gynecology*, question the effectiveness of antidepressant medications in actually relieving patients of their depressive symptoms.

Another huge drug group is the ADD, ADHD medications which have flooded the market and would lead us to believe we need them desperately to focus and accomplish a decent day's work.

From students who take **Adderall** to study, to **Concerta**, **Vyvanse**, and the good old **Ritalin**, more young and old are taking these drugs, which in fact, are nothing more than prescription speed. (**Adderall** is amphetamine salts.)

Bipolar Disorders

And finally, last, but certainly not least, is the recent epidemic of bipolar disorders that pretty much the entire world seems to suffer. Between **Abilify** and **Catapres** (an old antihypertension drug), along with antidepressants and other mood stabilizers, we have created a nation of walking zombies taking more medications instead of working out their problems or considering common-sense methods of treatment like diet, balancing hormones, exercise, and lifestyle to help with our increasing difficulties coping with our complicated lives.

On the topic of antidepressants I leave you with the following thought. If you are depressed or think you are not able to handle your life the way you believe you should, find a good therapist first and work hard to help yourself; only go to a psychiatrist if indeed the best course for you is to start medication. Use medication only temporarily, to get you over the bad times. Work with your doctor to help you discontinue taking antidepressants as soon as you can, before side-effects push you into taking more medications, or becoming more depressed. The problem with depression and other mood disorders is that the root cause is not a deficiency of these medications but often a hormone deficiency, a lifestyle issue, lack of sleep, bad diet, or an environmental problem (work, family, personal). Addressing your personal issues may accomplish a lot more than using medication and will certainly be a safer and more common-sense way to work at solving this immense issue with overmedication in our society.

Hot Flashes

Unfortunately, classical medical training offers only two options for treatment of hot flashes: synthetic/nonhuman identical hormone replacement (**Premarin, Prempro, Provera,** and **birth control pills**) and antidepressants (**Paxil, Zoloft, Effexor**). In the spring of 2013 the FDA approved a drug named **Brisdelle**, which is a low-dose **Paxil** specifically for the treatment of hot flashes.

The Multiple Advisor Problem

An outgrowth of our present health care system is that many people go to more than one doctor on a regular basis, be it conventional, alternative, and more often a combination of the two.

One physician no longer overlooks nor understands the whole patient. No one supervises and coordinates all your medications, supplements, vitamins, diet, and exercise. You carry dozens of diagnoses attended to by just as many specialists. Your health care is horribly fragmented and plain *bad*.

This situation shortchanges the patient and renders the doctor unable and often unwilling to help. Although difficult to accomplish, the onus is on you to make the doctor of your choice a true partner in your total health. If you can get organized, compassionate, objective information, you can start helping yourself and your doctor put the puzzle of your health care together. If you are afraid of your doctor and hold back information about medication and supplements you are taking or significant issues and habits in your life, you are only hurting yourself. If the doctor you go to doesn't like what you have to say or discourages you from choosing options you feel strongly about, just leave the doctor. You can always find a better doctor! It's a matter of life and death!

The medical literature is unclear on the way in which antidepressant medication works in the treatment of hot flashes. It appears to be a desperate attempt to offer some kind of relief to the patient in the absence of the real option that bioidentical/human identical hormones offer.

Of the thousands of patients I have seen with hot flashes, not one has stayed with **Zoloft** or **Paxil** longer than a few months when used for the treatment of hot flashes. The stories I hear are always the same. For the first few weeks, the medication seems to be helping, but then it stops and the doctor has to increase the dosage. With increasing dosage, serious side-effects arise while the flashes return and the patient and often the doctor just give up. In my opinion (and theirs), this is not a satisfactory method of combating one of the most troublesome symptoms of hormone imbalance.

Hot flashes are often treated with **Premarin**, **Megace** (in breast cancer patients), and **birth control pills**. Their alleged goal is to replace low estrogen levels believed to cause hot flashes. Their mode of action with respect to treatment of hot flashes is unknown. No research exists to substantiate a working mechanism for the relief of the symptoms. In my experience the side-effects from these therapies are so numerous, the level of dissatisfaction with the results so high, they nullify any benefits.

While **Premarin** and **birth control pills** do eliminate hot flashes, in many women they create significant breast tenderness, vaginal bleeding, weight gain, mood swings, and gastrointestinal discomfort. Not to mention the question of a potential increase in the risk of breast and uterine cancer. (See Chapter 9, Synthetic/Nonhuman Identical Hormones and Cancer.)

Quite ironically, since the 1970s, women in Europe have been placed on birth control pills through menopause to prevent hot flashes. In the U.S., this practice was considered bad medicine in the 1980s when women were taken off birth control pills by the time they reached age 35, regardless of fertility status.

Today, the American College of Obstetrics and Gynecology recommends women stay on birth control pills pretty much indefinitely through the menopausal transition. How these synthetic hormones that suppress our entire body's production of hormones are used with such impunity is beyond my understanding.

According to conventional gynecology, the controversy around **Premarin** and other synthetic/nonhuman identical estrogens in general makes the decision to take them to relieve hot flashes very difficult, yet **birth control pills**, which are pretty much the same, are considered safe and women are encouraged to use them indefinitely. Go figure.

Insomnia and Sleep Disorders

Although insomnia and sleep disorders are often caused by hormone imbalance, other agents can be culprits too. Stress, changes in environment, heavy meals late at night, a bed partner who snores, a bed partner you no longer want to share the bed with, shift work, jet lag, heavy exercise before bedtime, and drinking alcoholic or caffeinated beverages at night are all common causes of sleep problems. When a patient comes to the doctor's office and complains of insomnia, most physicians are not trained to even think of what may be causing the insomnia, let alone find the root cause of the problem. Most doctors usually take the easy way out and prescribe medications.

Most sleeping pills belong to the group of medications called hypnotics (sleep-inducing). The most commonly prescribed sleeping medications are **Ambien, Lunesta, Roserem, Restoril,** and **Sonata**. Another group of medications used to treat insomnia are benzodiazepines (also used to treat anxiety and panic attacks, as previously described). They include **Xanax, Valium, Klonopin,** and **Ativan**. Over-the-counter medications include **Excedrin PM, Tylenol Extra Strength PM, Nytol,** or **Unisom**. These formulations contain the same ingredient, diphenhydramine (**Benadryl**), an antihistamine that makes you drowsy, dries you up, may give you nightmares and certainly makes you a zombie the next day.

Although sleeping pills do help you fall asleep, the quality of sleep they induce is not natural. Users of these medications don't dream or have nightmares or disturbingly vivid dreams, since the drugs alter natural sleep patterns. REM (rapid eye movement) sleep is the most beneficial part of your sleep and sleeping pills eliminate it completely. As a result, people tend to be groggy the next day, they walk around in a fog, cannot concentrate, and their libido disappears over time with their extended usage.

Again, classical medicine teaches us to treat symptoms and not the root cause of insomnia and sleep disorders, creating a large population dependent on medication to fall asleep but never really finding the reasons and true solutions for their sleep problem.

Over the past 35 years I have written hundreds of prescriptions for sleeping pills and I continue today. If used judiciously, sparingly, and only when really needed, sleeping pills and sedatives will help with an occasional bout of insomnia in particularly stressful times, when traveling, or when hormone balance is just off. But, if you find yourself taking them every night and still not feeling well rested in the morning, stop and find out the root cause and try to fix that.

Look at your life, your hormone status, and find the real reasons for your problem with sleep because without a good night's sleep you won't be healthy for long. (Read more about sleep in Chapter 10.)

Headaches and Migraines

A visit to your conventional internist or primary care practitioner with the complaint of headaches will usually elicit one of two reactions. Either the physician will perform an examination and upon finding no abnormalities in your neurologic exam treat you with medications, or he/she will send you to a neurologist for a battery of diagnostic tests to rule out everything from a brain tumor to multiple sclerosis. Assuming you get a clean bill of health and your diagnosis is migraines or just headaches, the doctor will opt for medications before even asking you about your diet, exercise, hormone connection (like frequency around your periods), or sleep patterns.

The most commonly used prescription medications to treat migraines are **Relpax**, **Topamax**, **Amerge**, **Zomig**, **Maxalt**, **Imitrex** (tablets and injectable), **Fioricet**, **Depakote**, and **Inderal**.

Over-the-counter analgesics such as **Ibuprofen** and **Acetamino- phen** are also prescribed. Narcotic painkillers like **Percocet** and **Vicodin** or even **Oxycontin** are occasionally used as well. Many new drugs are now on the market that migraine specialists recom- mend to prevent migraines. Their side-effects are numerous and their effectiveness minimal at best.

In my practice, I find that most patients I treat for migraines respond well to **Fioricet**. As with all pharmaceuticals, the potential side-effects must always be considered. Stomach irritation, diar- rhea, dizziness, fainting, and skin rashes are most common.

Migraines are often treated with **Botox** these days and many patients and physicians swear by the great results they are getting.

Over-the-counter medications include all the nonsteroidal anti-inflammatory drugs (NSAIDs) such as **Motrin, Ibuprofen, Aleve, Advil,** and so on. Although their manufacturers would have you believe there are differences among them, they are all the same. **Tylenol** (acetaminophen) and all brands of aspirin (**Bayer, Excedrin**, and so forth) are occasionally effective in treating mild migraines. If you are taking over-the-counter medications and experience no significant improvement in your symptoms within 24 hours of taking the medications as prescribed, seek professional advice. You may have been given an incorrect diagnosis and may be taking the wrong medication. Be honest with yourself and take stock and make sure you are not suffering from a hangover, dehy- dration, a cold, sinus problems, are eating food to which you are allergic, or have neck problems or exercising too much.

Loss of Sex Drive/Loss of Libido

Loss of sex drive in women is seldom addressed by classical conven- tional medicine practitioners as it requires embarrassing personal disclosures many doctors do not feel comfortable with, thus leaving too many women to suffer thinking that there is something wrong with *them*, that they alone are suffering, leading to exacerbation of the problem. The only significant research in the area of sexual function comes from the 1960s by Masters and Johnson. Human sexuality is such an important topic it seems odd our studies are from more than 50 years ago. Sporadic articles appear in medical and psychiatric journals dealing with human sexuality, but as a rule, there are no mainstream publications to educate the doctors to help women and men who are suffering mostly in silence.

The growing concern for treatment of male impotence, commonly referred to as "erectile dysfunction," led to the FDA approval of **Viagra** (sildenfil) in 1999. **Viagra**, researched as an anti-hypertension medication, proved a bigger hit when its side-effect turned out to be stronger and longer erections in the men studied. Its mechanism of action is to increase blood flow to the pelvic area, meaning penis and vagina (so it does work on women as well). We all need significant increase in blood flow to our genital areas to get aroused and then actually have sex. Viagra does accomplish that, so from a mechanical standpoint it works. Unfortunately, having sex and feeling sexy are not the same. **Viagra, Cialis,** and **Levitra** make the act of sex mechanically easier but none of these drugs will help improve flagging hormone levels and stale relationships.

To date few studies have been published addressing female libido in aging women. The only promise is in the vaginal use of preparations of estradiol, estriol, testosterone, and DHEA (all bioidentical/human identical hormones). The new drug the FDA approved as the equivalent to Viagra (flibanserin) has no scientific data or clinical application to support its success. So doctors in clinical settings make their treatment decisions based on experience and often just discard the woman with a pat on the back and a condescending, "It's just part of aging, honey."

I don't believe this situation is acceptable.

Vaginal dryness may be a local symptom, but its cause is systemic and should be addressed with systemic treatment with bioidentical hormones. Women must no longer accept that aging goes along with loss of sex drive and dwindling sexuality, while it is acceptable for men to stay sexually active indefinitely.

In conclusion, conventional/classical medicine still addresses patient complaints from the standpoint of treatment with medications for the individual complaint in the context of a disease-focused philosophy. It rarely addresses the root cause of symptoms, specifically in the area of hormone imbalance. Use this chapter to keep you informed of what your conventional doctor knows. A good doctor-patient relationship will ensure the best outcome for you. So, nurture a partnership with your doctor and recommend he/she learn about hormones in wellness and disease prevention. You will both benefit greatly.

CHAPTER 5

Alternative Treatments for Symptoms of Hormone Imbalance

Alternative therapies have emerged over the course of the past two decades out of the public's dissatisfaction with the consistently poor performance of conventional/classical treatments. The classical medical system has boxed itself into only diagnosing and treating disease, is tightly bound to the FDA, and is totally dependent on medication usage rather than focusing on true prevention. Although attempts to change public perception have been made with a push for earlier diagnosis of disease with the help of mammography, colonoscopy, PAP smears, lipid profile measurement, bone density, and genetic testing, the obsession with diagnosing diseases has left conventional medicine unable to help people stay healthy. Conventional medicine is only useful for acute care and diagnosis of disease. Prevention and wellness are outside its scope.

What conventional medicine considers prevention, such as PAP smears, mammograms, colonoscopies, and cardiac stress tests, are methods of diagnosing diseases at earlier stages. Not one of these methods actually prevents diseases from occurring. Just take a moment and think about it. How do any of these tests prevent anything?

Alternative Treatments for Symptoms of Hormone Imbalance

Desperately aware of the need to prevent disease, the public has been searching for different avenues to true prevention. As we live longer and strive for healthier lives, postponing and slowing the aging process is rapidly becoming a must for an ever-growing number of people. In fact, multibillion-dollar alternative, holistic, anti-aging, integrative, functional, complimentary, orthomolecular, functional—all names for preventive medicine specialties—have sprouted and are highly successful and sought after. Premenopause, menopause, and andropause have fueled the anti-aging and preventive health industry. Billions of dollars are spent every year by people in search of alternative treatments.

While the alternative trend is booming, it behooves conventional doctors to stop downplaying the importance of alternative medicine, become knowledgeable in the options and thus stay true to the mission of helping the patients. Discarding information and modalities we have not been taught in school is not the way to help but rather to lose patients.

Medical training in the conventional world still discounts alternative options and discourages conventional doctors from seeking information. I had to do my own research and work with my patients to figure out how best to help them and myself. In the end, I became truly informed as I began to use alternative therapies in conjunction with conventional medicine in my practice with continuously improving and reassuring results. This chapter offers an overview of the alternative medicine world my patients and I have been using over the past two decades.

Before you try any of these remedies, I strongly suggest you seek real professional advice. Be careful and cautious about advice given by salespeople in health food stores, online advertising by marketers raving about the particular product they are selling, self-proclaimed gurus with no real training or experience, or media-savvy salespeople with the goal of making money off your fears and desperation. Stop falling prey to the hype of well marketed cure-all supplements. Just like with drugs, only seemingly less dangerous, you don't know what is in the capsule or tablet, you don't know what the effects of the promoted stuff will be, you don't know how they will interact with the medications you're taking. Pyramid schemes abound in the world of alternative medicine so—buyer beware. Find a caring physician interested in alternative therapies, go to a health care provider with experience and get the most knowledgeable help available.

Even though the products I write about in this chapter are available over-the-counter, they may not be as safe or as effective as we would like to believe they are. Remember, there is only one of you and every time you take a supplement or medication or food, you affect your entire body's balance. One fatal mistake is all you can make. Unfortunately, there are no statistics to tell us how many people get into trouble because they take supplements and prescribed drugs, because most patients do not tell their doctors the truth about the supplements and vitamins or medications they are taking out of fear of being belittled or dismissed.

Government Regulation of Supplements and Herbs

Most supplements and herbs are not regulated by the Food and Drug Administration (FDA).

FDA approval is a very expensive process reserved for wealthy pharmaceutical companies. Having obtained FDA approval, drug companies can make certain claims about their medications that allow them to charge higher prices for their products. Unfortunately, FDA approval does not guarantee safety or efficacy. It's part of a dangerous game where the bottom line, not the patient, matters the most.

However, in spite of a neverending list of FDA-approved fiascos, most people and conventional physicians are oddly still more comfortable with FDA-approved drugs than herbals or supplements and vitamins. And the media reinforce this stance by consistently reporting any negative issues with alternative products while omitting problems with FDA approved drugs. This situation leads the public to believe that FDA-approved drugs are safer even if that is not quite so.

Before we move on to the non-FDA-approved alternative options, I would like you to know one more thing. While I am a conventional physician and prescribe FDA-approved drugs every day, I know the FDA doesn't approve any drug for long-term usage. The role of the FDA is to approve drugs for short-term usage based on scientific data provided by the manufacturer of the drug. Once a drug is approved by the FDA and reaches the market, it is the responsibility of the drug manufacturer to report to the FDA any untoward effects. The longer a drug is on the market and the more it is used, the more likely we are to find out its true safety and efficacy record. The caveat being that it's the responsibility of the manufacturer to report problems. There is no oversight by the FDA and many drugs stay on the market longer then they should because if they make money there is little incentive for their manufacturer to report problems.

That's why in my practice I prefer to use old drugs with established safety track records with millions of users over many decades. So the next time your doctor offers you the newest drug sample to treat your allergies, blood pressure, or diabetes, consider opting for an older drug and skip being a guinea pig in the pharmaceutical game. It will serve you better in the long run.

Alternative Therapies

Supplements and vitamins are not under FDA supervision. According to The Dietary Supplement Health and Education Act (DSHEA) of 1994 a dietary supplement is a product that contains a "dietary/food source ingredient" intended to supplement the diet. Dietary ingredients include vitamins, minerals, herbs or other botanicals, amino acids and substances such as enzymes, organ tissues, glandulars, and metabolites. Dietary supplements can also be extracts or concentrates, and may be found in many forms such as tablets, capsules, softgels, gelcaps, liquids, or powders.

These products may make therapeutic claims but must be labeled by law to say, "These statements have not been evaluated by the Food and Drug Administration. This product is not intended to diagnose, treat, cure, or prevent any disease." Again, this does not mean that they are not safe or effective. All it means is the law states they must provide these labels. Nonetheless, this situation leaves us, the public, in a precarious position. Whenever you go to a health food store, you are buying on faith. (Not that when you buy FDA-approved you don't.)

The information on the label is often vague, mostly out of fear by the seller that the FDA will stop them from selling the product if it's associated with any significant curative claims. You will never know exactly what is in the pill you're taking and basically have to rely on marketing information, the internet, and friends' recommendations. And that's a scary thought. We live in a society where the best marketer, the company that spends the most money on advertising, the biggest celebrity, the most recognized face, gets products sold. Not that there is much of a difference between the situation with supplements and FDA-approved pharmaceuticals. Only difference is FDA-approved usually requires a prescription from a physician giving a sense of scientific credibility. The truth is we have no idea what either contains, but we do take them on faith in the hopes they will help.

So how do you choose which supplement or herb to take?

Who Is the Product Manufacturer?

When I started researching supplements, vitamins, and herbs used to treat symptoms of hormone imbalance, I learned something I subsequently discovered few people knew. Despite the enormous variety of brands that fill the shelves of our health food stores, our supplements, vitamins, herbs, skin creams, enzymes, and so on are mostly made by the same few companies. That means we are buying the same product packaged with different labels at different prices.

Let me explain a little further.

Let's take **Black Cohosh**, a herbal supplement that presumably improves hot flashes. Black Cohosh can be found in stores under as many as 20 different labels, **Remifemin** being the most popular. Most Black Cohosh is produced by a handful of manufacturers and then sold on the open market under a variety of brands. It is impossible to determine who the manufacturer is. Nowhere on the label does that information appear. Anybody can contract with not only the manufacturer but also with distributors (the middlemen) to put their own label on a supplement, and then sell it to the public. It's that simple.

This situation leaves the entire industry and the user in an uncomfortable position. In order to maintain credibility and safety and as more pharmaceutical companies have gotten involved in the nutraceutical business, they need laboratory testing and manufacturing to be at the same level as pharma standards. The products must be standardized. Standardized means that the dosing is consistent across all batches of the supplement or herb. For instance, **St. John's wort** made by Pharmanex has the same amount of active ingredients in every bottle labeled by Pharmanex. Since there is no regulatory agency that requires standardization of dosing, the manufacturer decides whether to provide internal testing and quality control for their products. In the preceding case, Pharmanex happens to be a pharmaceutical company with FDA-approved products and their supplements are pharmaceutical grade. Other large pharmaceutical companies around the globe have taken the lead and improved quality of supplement production, thus improving quality and standardization over the past decade as the industry has reached a trillion dollars in sales a year.

Please do not rush to buy the cheapest or the newest supplement endorsed by a celebrity or marketed on social media with the most dollars. If it sounds too good to be true, it is. Chances are it is just pie in the sky. Work with a doctor, a chiropractor, a naturopath, a specialist who really knows supplements and vitamins and who doesn't flood you with 50 pills a day because he is selling the product and stands to profit from it.

I advise you to stick with standardized products for your own safety. Since there are so many on the market, work with a real expert who knows more than one brand and is qualified and experienced who represents your best interests. This is where an integrative, holistic, conventionally trained physician is your best bet.

Bioavailability

Assuming you have chosen a reliable brand with a proven track record there still are no guarantees the supplement will work for you. A potential stumbling block to benefiting from your chosen herb, vitamin or supplement is bioavailability.

A big word with big implications, bioavailability means the amount of the active ingredient in the medication or supplement that gets into your bloodstream and can effectively be used by your body. You could take pounds of supplements without visible improvement in your condition simply because your body is unable to extract its beneficial ingredients. A perfect example is yam in its natural form. Although yams contain substances that can be metabolized into progesterone, the real hormone our body makes and needs, eating yams or slathering on yam creams or taking yam supplements will never give you the progesterone you need. That is because our bodies cannot turn yams into bioavailable progesterone.

How the drug or supplement gets into your system, what the body does with it once it's in your bloodstream, how much of it gets to your cells, and how they use it are only parts of the bio-availability story. When FDA-approved drugs are tested for effectiveness, the most important marker is their bioavailability (pharmacokinetics—how much gets into your blood stream and how long it stays there). With supplements and food substances, bioavailability is not often addressed. When it is, it becomes a marketing term rather than the proof of its usefulness to your body.

A perfect example of variable bioavailability in supplements is calcium. Calcium is essential to good bone structure and has been widely marketed as the supplement needed to keep our bones healthy. Even though we had no science to support the connection between taking oral calcium and preventing osteoporosis, we kept on taking and recommending more and more of it just because it was well marketed. But taking large quantities of calcium supplements does not ensure that more calcium gets into our system, let alone to our bone cells or into our bones. Let's follow the path of a calcium pill you take in the evening, three hours after your last meal or before bedtime. Your stomach is empty and the pill gets broken down into tiny fragments by gastric juices. If the fragments are small enough, the calcium supplement you took gets absorbed into your bloodstream. If it isn't small enough, it goes through the stomach and into the intestine and out the other end—no calcium for your body. If it's absorbed into your bloodstream it has a chance of getting to your bone cells. But once there, there is no guarantee that the cells that need the calcium have the enzymes, receptors, and other elements necessary to absorb the calcium molecules and then use them to keep your bones strong.

The path I use to describe the fate of calcium in your body is exactly the same as that for all food or medication you take. There are lots of great supplements available with incredible potential benefits. The reason they don't live up to their promises is because they are not bioavailable and your body just gets rid of them instead of using them to its benefit. This is one of the key reasons many supplements just don't work.

In an attempt to improve bioavailability, many manufacturers advise taking their supplements and some drugs (thyroid medication is a perfect example) on an empty stomach. The reason behind this method of administration is that hypothetically, an empty stomach will digest and absorb a supplement better than if mixed with other foods or medications. I stress *hypothetically*, because there are no studies to substantiate the bio-availability of most supplements on the market today.

So for now, I've learned to focus on the use of a few supplements manufactured by pharmaceutical grade labs under the Evolved Science (eshealth.com) label. The goals of the supplement line I have developed are: to increase energy, decrease inflammation, improve immune function and provide hormone support. The results speak for themselves.

The degree of bioavailability of a substance is directly proportional to its expected effect. If you are taking a pill to get rid of a headache and the headache is gone within an hour of taking the pill, clinically speaking, the pill was bioavailable enough to be considered effective. Now you know how we do it in our practice. Make sure the professional you work with does it the same way; it'll save you money and time. And you won't find yourself taking 50 pills a day and not knowing what they are supposed to do or if they are doing it.

Fatigue

Most men and women in middle age complain of fatigue as a primary reason for seeking help.

Getting up more tired than when you went to bed, poor quality sleep, and tossing and turning are a few of the problems leading to

Professional Advice

When taking herbal supplements, the type of professional advice you get is critical.

Because herbs and supplements are not prescription medications, millions of people just buy them without advice from a professional. That may feel like a freeing experience, but the risk of getting into trouble is very high, especially when you are taking other medications as well.

I am blessed with a group of highly intelligent and proactive patients. Whenever I ask them how they make their choices of supplements, the answers astound me—friends, TV ads, Dr. Oz, women's magazines, celebrity endorsements, and of course FB, other forms of social media, and the internet. Missing from this list is a real qualified expert. Mostly because there is a paucity of truly qualified experts. When you walk into a health food store, the salesperson is your resource and your expert in residence. When you go to an alternative doctor or naturopath, he/she will sell you supplements because they cannot write prescriptions for medications or hormones. Experts in alternative medicine don't know much about disease processes and conventional doctors don't know much about herbs and supplements (I'm being very generous when saying this). The world of supplements is a new frontier and although we glibly use dozens a day, we have little insight into their long-term effects, interactions or side-effects. So please be careful out there!

fatigue. Diseases labeled by alternative medical practitioners such as chronic fatigue and fibromyalgia give a nice label to unexplained fatigue but they don't mean much to the mainstream nor do they lead to reliable or consistent treatments.

Aging, poor diet, and medications with side-effects that block the body's ability to refresh and rejuvenate during a healthy sleep cycle compound the problem. Natural ways to help diminish fatigue include but are not limited to supplements like **L-carnitine** and **Coenzyme Q$_{10}$, caffeine, choline, inositol,** and herbals like

artichoke extract, green tea extract, Holy basil, ashwagandha root, ginseng, astragalus, certain mushrooms, maca, rhodiola, and vitamins B complex, D, and **NADH.**

Bloating

The action of herbal diuretics is milder than their pharmaceutical counterparts and they do not deplete your body's potassium or produce side-effects like acute gout, gall stones, kidney stones, or stomach problems.

Green Tea—Try two to three cups of green tea a day or green tea supplements. For people who can't tolerate caffeine, many try decaffeinated green tea or take natural caffeine-free supplements.

Dandelion Leaf—Dandelion leaf is one of the most effective herbal diuretics available. Dandelion leaf contains several essential minerals and vitamins, including potassium, which make it safer than a prescription diuretic.

Stinging Nettle—Stinging nettle leaf also contains several essential minerals including potassium, iron, and magnesium. It is available in tea, capsule, and tincture form. The only reported side-effect of stinging nettle leaf is stomach upset.

Yarrow—Yarrow is an effective diuretic also rich in flavonoids, minerals, and vitamins. It is available in tablet, capsule, extract, and tincture form as well as in tea form. People who are allergic to ragweed, aspirin, or who are already taking a medication for anxiety, insomnia, or high blood pressure should not use yarrow. Other herbs that may be effective as a diuretic include **Chickpea, Uva Ursi, Ginseng, Goldenseal, Parsley, Yellow Dock,** and **Celery.**

Always remember, you should tell your doctor you are taking herbal remedies if you also take prescription medications since they may interact. But also keep in mind your doctor isn't likely to know much about supplements and herbs and may either tell you to stop taking them or diminish their importance. Sadly, you are pretty much alone out there. Don't take your doctor's response as the gospel any more than your naturopath's say so.

While I do prefer conventional diuretics, I would never discourage a patient who wants to go the natural way from eating a few stalks of celery or drinking **a green drink with kale, ginger, lemon, spinach, celery, and green apple.** Just don't take them all together and pay attention to how you feel. Your body is never wrong. All you have to do is listen to its messages.

Postpartum Depression, General Depression, and Mood Swings

Relaxation techniques, meditation, yoga breathing, consistent sleep (minimum 7½ to 8 hours a night), lots of water (preferably alkaline, ph>8.5) and a diet low in processed foods (no canned or bagged foods from a shelf in the supermarket), low in carbohydrates (no breads, pasta, rice, potato, or desserts), high in polyphenols (berries of all kinds), and no alcohol (no matter how many studies to the contrary, alcohol wreaks havoc on our system, making us age faster) will all help improve mood. In addition, there are a few herbals and supplements that may also help. There are no studies comparing dependency on conventional versus alternative antidepressants or efficacy so anyone who discounts your idea of trying supplements has no scientifically sound basis for discouraging you.

Fish Oil

Fish oil is rich in omega-3 and omega-6 fatty acids, scientifically proven building blocks supporting optimal brain chemistry, antioxidants and hair, joints, and nail support. Although Americans seem to get adequate amounts of omega-6 fatty acids from nuts, we often come up short in omega-3s, which are most readily available in cold-water fish (salmon, trout, herring, sardines, mackerel, tuna, and swordfish). Without enough omega-3s, nerve signals aren't transmitted properly in the brain, leaving us depressed or anxious. A 2007 study of 43 adults found that those with diets high in omega-6s but low in omega-3s had high levels of pro-inflammatory cytokines, which are molecules that tend to be produced in the body when people are depressed or stressed. One 2009 study found that higher intakes of omega-3s and oily fish may reduce the number of depressive episodes in women by about 30 percent.

Some people report an unpleasant aftertaste or "fish burps" after taking omega-3 and omega-6 fish oils. This usually can be avoided by making sure your fish oil is made from "clean," pollutant-free (mercury-free) fish, and even refrigerating or freezing the supplement. Make sure your supplement contains both EPA and DHA. At Evolved Science (eshealth.com) we work with 2,000–4,000 mg/day combinations with excellent results. All you have to remember is that fish oils affect bleeding parameters (like aspirin, only safer), so if you are having any kind of surgery, even minimal (e.g., cosmetic or dental), you want to discontinue their use for the week before and after surgery.

B-Complex Vitamins

One of common culprits for mild depression and low thyroid function may be an imbalance of brain neurotransmitters, natural chemicals that can act as mood enhancers by enhancing signal transmission among brain cells. Prescription antidepressants like Prozac and other selective serotonin reuptake inhibitors (SSRIs) focus on one of these neurotransmitters in particular, serotonin, which they allow to stay around longer in the system as previously addressed. A more natural solution is supplementing with vitamins B_6 and B_3 (niacinamide). These vitamins make your body conserve the amino acid tryptophan and convert it to serotonin.

A 2004 Danish study of 140 people found that those who were clinically depressed had low levels of vitamin B_6 in their blood.

If upping serotonin levels through B_6 and B_3 doesn't help, the problem might be a deficiency of some of the other neurotransmitters in the brain like norepinephrine and dopamine. Vitamin B_{12} and folic acid are two supplements necessary for the synthesis of these two hormones. A 2002 Dutch study of nearly 4,000 elderly people found that many of those who had depression symptoms also had vitamin B_{12} deficiencies.

So instead of opting for antidepressants for PMS, postpartum depression, and general depression, adding a regimen of B_{12}, B_6, and B_3 to bioidentical hormones may be a safer and easier option.

5-HTTP: An amino acid, 5-hydroxytryptophan, or 5-HTP (a serotonin precursor), is a natural option for raising serotonin levels. If absorbed, 5-HTP is converted into serotonin in the body and unlike SSRIs (the antidepressants with all their side-effects), 5-HTP may increase the amount of serotonin we make. A six-week study of 63 people found that those who took 300 mg 5-HTP daily had the same depression relief as those who took prescription antidepressants but with fewer side-effects. 5-HTP may cause loose stools so taking it in an oil base is easier to absorb and may prevent stomach issues.

L-Theanine: This is an amino acid derivative found in green tea. L-theanine has long been known to trigger the release of gamma-aminobutyric acid (GABA) in the brain. GABA activates the major calming neurotransmitters, promoting relaxation and reducing anxiety, but the body has difficulty absorbing supplements containing synthesized GABA. We have been using L-theanine in our practice for more than five years with great results. Patients report feeling calmer, less anxious and able to focus clearly. All this without side-effects or dependency.

Vitamin D: While initially considered only useful in maintaining healthy bones because it promotes calcium absorption, vitamin D is in fact a hormone. It helps combat anxiety and depression while also protecting from cancer and helping other hormone production and improving general hormone balance. A 2008 study of 441 overweight and obese men and women in Norway found that those given 20,000 and 40,000 IUs vitamin D3 per week significantly felt improvement in mood and diminished depression after one year as opposed to a placebo group. It's unclear how vitamin D diminishes depression but then we still don't know how the entire list of FDA-approved antidepressants work either.

Concerns about vitamin D toxicity are limited. In our practice, we follow vitamin D levels with routine blood tests. The most popular form of vitamin D supplementation in our practice is a liquid form of the active form D3. (For more on our vitamins visit www.eshealth.com.)

St. John's Wort

Extracts of this herb have been used in folk medicine for hundreds of years. In Germany, St. John's wort is licensed for the treatment of anxiety, depression, and sleep disorders. The extracts that make up this remedy contain many different chemical classes, so the "active agent" is unknown. The use of St. John's wort extracts to treat mild to moderate depression is supported by numerous clinical studies. Its efficacy is comparable to standard tricyclic antidepressants but without the severe side-effects. Therapeutic response occurs in days to weeks with minimum treatment duration of four to six weeks in any reported study. Side-effects include fatigue, allergic reactions, and stomach discomfort but no long-term dependency.

SAMe

An amino acid supplement, S-adenosylmethionine (ah-de-no-sil meh-thio-neene) has been used by some psychiatrists in the treatment of depression, for more than 20 years, predominantly in Europe. Claims in the treatment of osteoarthritis, liver disease, fibromyalgia and chronic pain have been made in the popular literature over the past 12 years. The problem with SAMe is that dosing is critical and unless taken under the supervision of a knowledgeable practitioner, low doses yield limited results, the patient becomes discouraged and discontinues it. The over-the-counter recommended dosage for SAMe is significantly less than the dosage needed for optimum results, making it potentially unsafe for a patient to self-medicate to reach desired outcome based on Internet search data.

When using alternative antidepressants in my practice, I find mixed results. The cost of the medication often becomes prohibitive at the doses patients require to feel significant improvement. Consistently we find the use of human identical/bioidentical hormones, balancing the thyroid and adrenal, dietary changes, exercise, and talk therapy provide substantial improvement in mood, minimizing the need for either conventional or alternative antidepressants.

Hot Flashes

In Chapter 4, we learned that conventional medicine has various hormone preparations to offer for the treatment of hot flashes.

Doing my own research over the course of more than 5 years I permanently settled on natural/bioidentical/human identical hormones as the safest and most effective option for treatment of hot flashes in my practice by 2000.

Black Cohosh, Vitex, and **Oil of Evening Primrose** are the most popular herbal supplements in this category. Over the years I have found women swear by these supplements, while others find them totally useless. Consistently when hot flashes increase in frequency and other symptoms of hormone depletion compound the picture, herbal remedies become less effective.

Black Cohosh: Its primary application is to help ease the physical and mental changes associated with perimenopause and menopause such as hot flashes, headaches, irritability, and depression. Black Cohosh has been used to symptomatically treat hormonal deficits arising from ovariectomy and hysterectomy in younger women. While some clinical studies do exist to support the primary use of Black Cohosh for the treatment of perimenopausal symptoms such as hot flashes, headaches, palpitations, ringing in the ears, sleep disturbances, and mood disorders, its mode of action is poorly understood. Treatment requires at least eight weeks to alleviate symptoms. Clinical studies have ranged from eight weeks to six months; the results are equivocal at best. Side-effects include stomach irritation, nausea, and dizziness. Although the supportive literature on Black Cohosh states that it can be used in conjunction with estrogen supplementation without side-effects I do not recommend it. Once on hormone supplementation, I see no reason to add supplements to relieve the symptoms hormones eliminate anyway.

Vitex: (Also known as chasteberry, monk's pepper, agnus castus, agni casti fructus, chaste tree.) This has more than one active ingredient, including flavonoids and iridoids. Some clinical data exist to support the use of Vitex extract in infertility associated with corpus luteum insufficiency, PMS and PMTS (premenstrual tension syndromes), acne especially associated with PMS, amenorrhea (lack of periods), polymenorrhea (too frequent periods), and mastodynia (breast discomfort). Most of the research on this product so far has been in Germany; results have led to the belief that Vitex acts on the anterior pituitary, decreasing prolactin levels and increasing progesterone levels. Vitex seems to improve the hormone balance and may temporarily relieve symptoms.

Although its use is widespread, the side-effects are quite limiting. They include diarrhea, weight gain, rashes, nausea and headaches. Vitex should not be used in combination with hormone treatment, birth control pills or while breast feeding.

Oil of Evening Primrose: Classified as an essential nutrient, evening primrose contains essential fatty acids (EFAs), particularly omega-6 and gamma linoleic acid (GLA). Used for skin disorders and hyperactivity in children, oil of evening primrose has found a great niche in women's health: PMS, breast health, pregnancy, lactation, and hair and nails support. Although often prescribed for symptoms of menopause, oil of evening primrose alone is of limited value in the treatment of hot flashes. I must also caution you that seizures have been reported in patients on antipsychotic medications who took oil of evening primrose with their medication (Internal Medicine, May 2001, "Alternatives Ease Some Menstrual Symptoms").

Insomnia and Sleep Disorders

Long before we had sleeping pills, herbal remedies were routinely used in the treatment of sleep disorders. Herbs are currently used for the treatment of insomnia not only in alternative practices, but in conventional ones as well.

Valerian: Also known as vandal root and garden heliotrope, Valerian finds its application in the treatment of insomnia, nervousness, and improvement of sleep quality and has been used in Europe for hundreds of years. A number of clinical trials have shown Valerian to be an effective sedative, with an efficacy comparable to standard prescription medications such as benzodiazepines (Valium). Valerian extracts generally display fewer side-effects than standard sleep medications, are better tolerated and present a lower risk of dependency. Chronic use may result in headache, excitability, insomnia, and irregularities in heartbeat not unlike conventional medications.

Kava: Used as a muscle relaxant and anti-anxiety herb, Kava has a significant sedative component. It has been used safely in Polynesian society for centuries. In European phytomedicine it is recommended for the treatment of mild insomnia, anxiety, and muscular tension. Some clinical studies have demonstrated that Kava induces a state of relaxation and calm without interfering with cognition, memory, or alertness.

Side-effects are rare and associated with excess use. They include skin rashes and a syndrome (a collection of symptoms) similar to Parkinsonism. After discontinuation of the medication, the symptoms eventually disappear. But who would like these symptoms anyway?

Melatonin: A hormone secreted by the pineal gland, melatonin has captured the public's attention because of its alleged effects on mood, sleep, and jet lag. Promoted as a miracle supplement, this hormone is available without prescription in over-the-counter dosing that varies from less than 1 mg up to 5 mg. It was the number one over-the-counter sleeping pill a decade ago when a book was written about it.

Unfortunately, its track record has been spotty. Study after study has failed to substantiate the claims made that melatonin is a perfect natural sleep remedy. Scientific and public health concerns over the disconnect between its wide use and evidence of benefit led to the convening of a workshop on melatonin by the National Institutes of Health in 1996. The workshop's general conclusions were that, while there have been no medical catastrophes caused by melatonin, no long-term positive effects have been identified either. Melatonin might be of benefit for people with sleeping disorders or travelers crossing multiple time zones used to lessen jet lag, but that seems to be an individual opinion rather than a scientific fact.

Since there are no negatives known with the usage of melatonin my position is that if my patients who take it think it helps, they should continue doing so. No one has reported sleep walking or having problems using heavy machinery when using melatonin. But some have reported vivid dreams.

A Word of Caution When it Comes to Herbal Supplements and Soy Derivatives

Black cohosh, isoflavones, ipriflavones, soy derivatives, soy milk, soy nuts, edamame, Vitex, and Dong Quai are phytoestrogens. Their chemical make-up resembles human estrogen molecules closely enough for the body to misread them as estrogens. For that reason, they seem to alleviate some of the symptoms of estrogen deficiency. But they are not estrogens and they do not offer the beneficial effects we obtain from estradiol—the natural/human identical estrogen. No research data to substantiate beneficial estrogen-like effects on the heart, bones or brain exist. In fact, there are many questions about negative effects from their long-term use.

Thus, while these soy derivatives may help reduce the discomfort associated with symptoms of estrogen deficiency, we may be doing ourselves a greater disservice. Heart disease, deterioration of our organ systems, and osteoporosis progress unimpeded when we take phytoestrogens.

The entire soy story comes from the fact that Japanese women in general don't suffer with symptoms of menopause. Japanese diet is rich in soy products from tofu, soy milk, and edamame. Hence, Japanese women don't suffer with menopausal symptoms because they eat lots of soy. This connection made by smart marketers made billions for the soy industry.

No scientific data supports this theory. Maybe it is genetics. Possibly Japanese women are genetically programmed to suffer fewer effects of hormone loss.

For now, I emphatically advise against the supplements isoflavones, ipriflavones, and genistein, available in capsules, powders, and gelcap forms. This does not mean you should stay away from soy milk, tofu, edamame, or other soy products. Soy in moderation is an excellent source of protein and its use should be limited to just that.

GABA: (Gamma Aminobutyric Acid) This is a naturally occuring amino acid with a significant inhibitory neurotransmission role in the brain. It acts as the body's calming mechanism and small studies reveal its effectiveness improving mood and helping relaxation and better sleep quality.

Headaches and Migraines

Alternative treatments for headaches include acupuncture, yoga, relaxation, meditation, breathing, massages, aromatherapy, and essential oils. Many patients shy from herbal remedies because of potential allergies that often worsen the headaches and interfere with the conventional medications they take.

Over time some supplements have gained acceptance for the treatment and even prevention of headaches.

Fish Oil: (Omega-3 and Omega-6) Enthusiasts and some scientific data demonstrate that fish oil reduces inflammation and works by reversing blood vessel dilation that often causes a headache. Even the conventional world has jumped onto the fish oil bandwagon, producing the FDA-approved version known as **Lovaza**. Just make sure you take good quality and the right dose.

Peppermint Oil: No conventional scientific data exist to support its use. However, there are no negative side-effects reported so trying it is unlikely to hurt you. It is used as a topical rub to the area of the head that experiences the most pain. Aromatherapy practitioners use it with reportedly good success.

Ginger: Whether in capsule or raw form, ginger is recommended by many alternative practitioners. No one knows how it works but there are no reported problems with it and it may reduce nausea associated with migraines.

Magnesium: A well-known and significant ingredient of our own bodies, its use as a supplement has been extensively studied. When taken in doses of 400 to 600 milligrams per day in oral formulations it is effective for migraines associated with auras and menstruation.

Magnesium may cause diarrhea if taken in large doses but is successfully used to decrease constipation and induces smooth muscle relaxation as well. In hospital settings magnesium is used extensively in preeclampsia (blood pressure elevation during the third trimester of pregnancy, during labor and delivery, necessitating treatment) and other acute medical problems, thus making it safe to use in prevention.

Vitamin B$_2$ (Riboflavin): Riboflavin can also act as a preventive of migraines. Studies have supported its use and other than sometimes making urine yellow or neon-colored, it doesn't cause any problems.

Coenzyme Q$_{10}$: One of the most important and ubiquitous enzymes, Coenzyme Q$_{10}$ is often helpful in high doses of up to 300 milligrams per day in reducing headaches. Directly involved in energy production at the cellular level CoQ$_{10}$ is crucial in the treatment of patients on statins, which severely deplete Coenzyme Q$_{10}$ and cause energy depletion and muscle spasms.

Butterbur: A most effective "natural medicine" in the treatment of headaches and migraines is butterbur. Butterbur is a plant grown in Germany, and studies have shown that in pill form it is effective in treating migraine pain and asthma, as well as alleviating upset stomachs. Butterbur is safe, but can only be ordered online since health food stores don't usually carry it.

Dong Quai: Although its main application is in the treatment of menstrual disorders and menstrual cramps, Dong Quai is often used to treat headaches. While there are practically no clinical studies on this herb, animal and *in vitro* studies suggest that Dong Quai may be useful as an anti-inflammatory, a smooth muscle relaxant, an analgesic, and a mild sedative.

Feverfew: This is often used in the prevention and treatment of migraines. The current consensus is that feverfew may work prophylactically to prevent migraines, and that emphasis should be placed on the use of high quality preparations with detectable and consistent levels of its key components (parthenolide levels of 0.2 percent to 0.9 percent). While clinical investigations have shown mixed results, two studies indicate that feverfew treatment results in a reduction in frequency of migraines and milder migraines in pretreated individuals. Feverfew in combination with vitamin B12 and magnesium appear to be associated with some decrease in frequency of headaches. Side-effects include stomach problems, diarrhea, allergic reactions to the fresh leaf when ingested, flatulence, and unpleasant taste.

Loss of Sex Drive and Loss of Libido

DHEA

Dehydroepiandrosterone (Di-hidro-epi-andro-sterone)—This is a precursor of testosterone and estradiol. It is available over-the-counter and many women use it to help improve sex drive. Data on the efficacy of DHEA vary. Improvement in sexual function may occur but side-effects of increased hair growth and acne limit the doses for optimum use. Scientific studies conducted and the use of DHEA in vaginal tablets or suppositories hold promise in the area of increasing libido. In our practice, for more than a decade, we have been using a combination of DHEA and estriol vaginal tablets with great success to increase libido and maintain vaginal lining integrity.

Another use for DHEA appears to be improvement of immune function, which becomes very important with the aging process. Data are still pending although DHEA has found a solid following in the conventional world of IVF and gynecological sex medicine.

CHAPTER 6

Natural/Bioidentical/Human Identical Hormones

As symptoms of hormone imbalance start increasing, most women try to ignore them. We justify them by thinking, "I'm too young," "This isn't really happening," "It'll just pass," or "I'll just do it the natural way." But the symptoms become more intense and difficult to handle. New symptoms crop up every day. Denial becomes impossible. We have to get help or just give up, get old and sick and buy larger clothes. Fear of cancer from hormones that started with the WHI study is still there and too many uninformed gynecologists still scare women away from getting help from hormones. Or even worse, they give them birth control pills, IUDs with synthetic hormones and antidepressants along with sleeping pills. As we've seen in previous chapters, initially, most women wind up treating the individual symptoms. This approach is the result of advice from professionals and lay people alike. At times, the treatment may seem successful. By taking this route, however, you quickly reach a point where you could be taking up to 50 pills a day—medications, herbs, and supplements—with limited success and much unintended and unsuspected interaction.

And not only because there are so many pills to take, so much fear and confusion, but above all, because they just don't work. As you get older, no matter how much research you do, how well you keep up with information, how organized and regimented in your exercise, lifestyle and diet routines, the outcome is consistently disappointing. Whether you chose alternative or conventional therapies, or integrate them both, at the end of the day you just don't feel like your old self anymore, life is starting to be uncomfortable and fear of getting old and sick becomes the overriding emotion.

No matter how hard you try to avoid using hormones, how much you try to diet, exercise and follow all lifestyle adjustments you know will help, without the help of bioidentical hormones, without the help of a little thyroid, a little adrenal support, you fall short. You cannot follow the diet because of cravings. You cannot exercise because you are too tired, your joints hurt, and you get easily injured. You cannot sleep and that leads to permanent exhaustion and brain fog. Your mood makes it impossible for you to get along with your loved ones, and even yourself, no matter how hard you try. You see, without hormones, it just doesn't work. Hormones open the door to feeling better and then all the pieces of the puzzle that you add to improve and maintain your health (proper nutrition, exercise, sleep, stress management, supplements, and so on) fall into place perfectly.

I have been caring for patients for more than 35 years, and I have suffered and experienced the devastation hormone deficiencies bring. Without fail, in every patient, myself included, I have found that without incorporating the proper balance of natural/bioidentical hormones, other treatments fall short and are essentially ineffective in the long run. In a vacuum, individually used, neither the conventional nor alternative therapies are capable of restoring your hormone balance or for that matter your best health. They may help alleviate symptoms temporarily, but if the root cause of your problems is hormone imbalance, measures that address only the symptoms will not help for long.

Georgia was 34 when she first came to see me. She had been going from doctor to doctor since she was 18. Her story was sad and all too common. When she turned 15 she got her period and with the beginning of her cycles, her life changed. She had terrible cramps, heavy bleeding, migraine headaches, and severe bloating. And her periods were irregular to boot. Her mother took her to the family doctor. Advil for the cramps, Imitrex for the headaches, and bed rest for the first day of her cycle were the doctor's advice.

A few years later, Georgia, then a college student, frustrated by the constant nuisance caused by her periods in spite of good diet, exercise, and Advil, went to see a gynecologist. This time she had a work-up: bloods, a physical examination, and a pelvic ultrasound. As you might have guessed, the results were all normal. Without hesitation, the doctor gave Georgia a prescription for birth control pills while at the same time diagnosing Georgia's problems as caused by hormone imbalance. After six months on the pill, things got worse. Her cramps were gone, her bleeding much lighter, but the migraines became incapacitating, the bloating unbearable, weight gain, and PMS unmanageable.

Georgia went to headache specialists, endocrinologists, and even joined Weight Watchers. Nothing worked. At 34, after 16 years of suffering, Georgia came to see me. I took Georgia off birth control pills and some of her symptoms (bloating, mood swings, and brain fog) improved within the first month. The headaches weren't as incapacitating, but her periods were heavy and lasted an entire week. After checking her hormone levels in the blood on the 17th day of her cycle two months after Georgia stopped taking birth control pills, once her system returned to normal I placed her on natural/bioidentical hormones (progesterone and a low-dose estradiol) and her symptoms vanished within a month.

Vanessa came to me at the age of 39. She had a long traumatic history of hormone imbalance. Not unlike Georgia, she too had painful, heavy periods, migraines, and PMS. But Vanessa learned to live with them and never went to a doctor. When she entered her mid-30s her bleeding pattern became erratic and even heavier. She finally saw a gynecologist. An ultrasound taken in the doctor's office revealed a large fibroid in her uterus (a benign tumor which does not turn into cancer but whose growth is connected to hormone imbalance and symptoms like heavy irregular bleeding and cramps). Vanessa was anemic and tired of bleeding. Her gynecologist suggested a hysterectomy and oophorectomy—and without much discussion Vanessa agreed. She was almost 40, had no plans to have children, and she knew that women without children had a higher incidence of ovarian cancer, so she asked the surgeon to just take everything out and get it all over with in one fell swoop.

The surgeon was all too happy to oblige. Lo and behold, within hours after the hysterectomy and oophorectomy (often known as total hysterectomy), Vanessa started experiencing hot flashes followed by night sweats, and then came the weight gain and severe depression. The doctor never mentioned that the surgery would throw her into menopause or that unless she received hormones she would feel worse than she did before the surgery. In the recovery room she had her first hot flash. Things went downhill from there. She was so desperate when she came to see me, she would have done anything to get her uterus and ovaries back along with her bad periods too. She's not alone. Too many doctors don't warn desperate women of the disastrous consequences of removing the organs that manufacture the hormones we need to survive. Maybe it's because our conventional medical training doesn't address the immediate and dramatic aftermath of hormone drop when surgery is performed, or worse, maybe they just don't care.

A few months after I placed Vanessa on natural/bioidentical/ human identical hormones in addition to thyroid and adrenal support, she did regain the hormone balance she literally could not live without, her life became normal again but to this day she is still sorry she allowed the surgical procedure and conducts seminars for women warning them of the association between hysterectomies and oophorectomies and traumatic postsurgical menopause. She is passionate about teaching women to question every physician recommendation, that women never get bullied or lulled into believing surgery has no consequences, and that the phrase "Everything will be fine, honey" is totally unacceptable under any circumstances. To date, Vanessa says, she has prevented thousands of women from unnecessary hysterectomies and I am honored to count her among my patients.

Connie was 66. She did not even remember her last period. Her doctor had told her she did not need to take any hormonal medications when she went through menopause. He was against synthetic hormone replacement in the wake of the results of the WHI study and like most traditionally trained gynecologists he thought bioidentical hormones would be of no use to her. He offered her a reminder to have annual PAPs and mammograms. Connie braved it through the first five years of menopause. She hardly survived the hot flashes, night sweats, and the total loss of sex drive. Eventually she could no longer stand getting old; her bones were thinning, she became wrinkled, her skin was thinning, and her joints were painful and stiff all the time. She woke up more tired than when she went to sleep and spent half the night tossing and turning and going to the bathroom. Her life was unbearable.

Stomach problems abounded. She was full of gas, bloated, and heartburn after every meal and during the night made her life hell. She gained 20 pounds, mostly around her middle section, and felt like a blimp. She became depressed. She couldn't bear looking in the mirror. She wanted more out of life and wasn't ready to throw in the towel. She went back to her doctor and three others. No doctor wanted to put her on hormones because they told her she was too old and the WHI study had made it clear that old women should not take hormones, of any kind. They offered her sleeping pills, antidepressants, diet pills, and told her to improve her diet and exercise regimens.

She got angry. The quality of her life was so poor she came into my office and told me that she would rather die than continue the path of deterioration she was on. I heard her. We spent a lot of time talking and did blood tests and biomarkers to find out the physiologic status of her heart, lungs, brain, and body composition. She was a normal aging woman who was suffering. She was at a crossroad. I could help her or I could let her go and she would slide down the slippery slope of chronic illness and incapacitating aging. I opted to help her and started her on natural/bioidentical/human identical hormones (estradiol and progesterone) in very low doses and built her up to where her symptoms improved, then I added thyroid to her regimen. She came to see me and said she "felt miraculously better." Her blood tests did not show significant levels of hormones. After all, the WHI did not study 17-beta estradiol, which is what bioidentical estrogen is, so the results of the study just did not apply nor did it provide help to this desperate woman who represents millions just like her.

Two years later, on her 68th birthday, 20 pounds lighter, sleeping eight uninterrupted hours a night, without aches and pains, and having sex again, Connie had become an outspoken proponent of giving women another chance with the support of the correct combination of bioidentical/human identical hormones she had found.

Don't get me wrong. There is no magic pill or cream solution, there are many pieces that interact and intertwine to bring health and youthful existence back. In her case her youthful appearance and general well-being were the results of natural/bioidentical/human identical hormones along with thyroid and adrenal supplementation, changes in her diet, consistent and correct exercise routines, and supplements I had first prescribed two years before but then tweaked as time went by. Hormones are the only solution to problems caused by hormone loss. Not a miracle, not witchcraft, not snake oil, not something new, simply scientifically sound, safe, and proven medical treatment that has been around in Europe and the U.S. for more than six decades.

What Are Natural/Bioidentical/Human Identical Hormones?

Natural, also known as bioidentical or better yet, human identical hormones are synthetically manufactured hormone drugs that look identical to the human hormone molecules our bodies make. These hormones are made from soy and yam oils by pharmaceutical processes of concentration and purification that produce hormone powders. These powders are then placed in different preparations for us to take (pills, patches, gels, lozenges, creams, and pellets).

Because these hormones look identical to our own hormones—estradiol, progesterone, testosterone, thyroid, growth hormone, insulin—I believe a better way to identify them is to call them human identical hormones to distinguish them from other hormone molecules that do not look like the hormones our bodies make. Short of human hormones, natural/bioidentical hormones are the closest in molecular structure, actions and interaction to our own hormones.

All hormones are synthetic because they are made in a lab but if their formula looks like the one of our own hormones they are known as bioidentical or natural in the world of prevention and estradiol, progesterone, testosterone, dessicated thyroid, compounded thyroid and human growth hormone in the conventional world. They are all the same.

Synthetic versus Natural Hormones

Very often you will hear conventional physicians tell you all hormone preparations are synthetic and there is no difference among them. The first part of that statement is correct. All hormone preparations are made in a laboratory. Regardless of whether they are made from plants or raw chemicals they are synthetic, meaning they are man-made. Hormones, unless taken directly out of the human body, are not human.

Synthetic doesn't mean bad. It just refers to the process of creating specific molecules in a laboratory, in this case, hormones.

In the case of bioidentical hormones, they are made from the oils of soy and yams that are plants, thus they were given the name "natural." However, no matter how much soy or yam you eat or slather on your body, it won't turn into the estrogen or progesterone inside your body.

To transform these plant oils into usable hormones we need pharmaceutical manufacturing processes. The products created are fine powders made of hormone molecules identical to the hormones our bodies make: estradiol, progesterone, and testosterone. These are what we call bioidentical/natural/human identical hormones.

All hormone preparations are synthetic because they are made in a pharmaceutical laboratory. All hormone preparations do not act the same in the human body.

Bioidentical or human identical hormones are recognized by the human body as our own and no adverse reactions to the hormones occur if when treating humans we follow the individual person's needs for hormones carefully and respectfully.

That is not the case with other hormone preparations like conjugated equine estrogens (Premarin), medroxyprogesterone acetate (Provera), and others, including birth control pills. These are the hormone preparations commonly referred to as synthetic hormones by the alternative medical groups.

These products are hormone impostors and they do not look anything like the hormone molecules our bodies make. They stop our own hormone production (in the case of birth control pills) or replace the hormones we need at perimenopause and menopause (Premarin and Provera). The body's reaction to these substances is totally different than the reaction to bioidentical or natural hormones. Our bodies do not like these substances and often react to them negatively.

Most cells that make up the organs in our body contain receptors, areas where, like a lock and key, hormones attach to the cell and do their jobs. While bioidentical/natural or human identical hormones fit perfectly into the specific hormone receptors on our cells, nonhuman identical hormones don't. It's like placing a round peg into a square hole. The receptors where the hormone molecules are supposed to fit change shape, change activity, and this mismatch creates both short- and long-term potentially dangerous effects. This phenomenon does not occur with bioidentical hormones; it only occurs with Premarin, Provera, and birth control pills.

The message is simple.

▶ All hormone preparations are synthetic because they are manufactured in a laboratory.

▶ Not all hormone preparations act the same in the human body.

▶ Nonhuman identical hormone preparations like Premarin (conjugated equine estrogen, ethinyl estradiol, and so on), Provera (medroxyprogesterone acetate, norethisterone, and so on), and birth control pills do not act the same as bioidentical/human identical hormones. (They have negative and very different effects on heart, cholesterol, blood clotting mechanisms, cancer growth, mood, brain function, and so forth.)

▶ Bioidentical or natural hormones fit into our body's receptors just like our own hormones do and provide us with the balance needed to keep us healthy and hormonally fit.

▶ Hormones that aren't bioidentical/human identical **replace** our hormones while bioidentical/natural/human identical hormones **supplement** our hormones.

The Effects of Natural/Biodentical Hormones On the Human Body

Because they are so similar in structure to our own body's sex hormones, the action of natural/bioidentical hormones when properly prescribed in the correct preparations is gentle and effective.

Natural Estrogen and Progesterone

Natural Progesterone, commonly referred to and known by the conventional and alternative medical communities as micronized progesterone, has the same chemical formula as the normally occurring sex steroid progesterone. Short of human progesterone, unavailable on the market, micronized progesterone is the next best thing. Because its chemical formula is the same as that of human progesterone, its actions are similar as well. Results are remarkable.

Human identical/Bioidentical Estrogens. 17-beta estradiol is the hormone made from soy and yam oils by chemical processes of concentration and purification in pharmaceutical laboratories. Its chemical molecular formula is the same as that of estradiol manufactured by the human body.

Scientific literature and extensive research on estrogens over the course of almost a century have shown that the most useful and safe estrogen is **estradiol. Estriol**, the estrogen most prevalent during pregnancy, may have some mild positive effect on keeping vaginal walls and skin moisturized but that the effect is limited and poorly studied. A study that looked at using estriol in multiple sclerosis failed to produce any significant results.

In some alternative treatments, combinations of estradiol with estriol and/or estrone are being promoted by compounding pharmacies and alternative physicians without scientific data to support safety or efficacy for these formulations (**Biest** and **Tri-Est**). Please avoid using them.

Many over-the-counter products include the name *natural* and *progesterone* on the label. Too often these labels only serve to confuse. Most of them contain yam creams and other supplements and vitamins as well as herbs but no real hormones. They are not the same products in the same concentrations as the natural estrogen (estradiol) and progesterone we are discussing in this chapter. Our bodies do not have the enzymes and chemical pathways necessary to transform soy or yams into usable hormones. (See Chapter 5, phytoestrogens and bioavailability).

The Difference Between Synthetic and Natural Hormones

In Chapter 4, we addressed conventional medical treatments for individual symptoms of hormone deficiency or imbalance. When hot flashes start, conventional medicine introduces synthetic estrogens. You now know that the term synthetic does not distinguish among types of hormones. It's how the hormone molecule looks that determines its action in the body.

To make safe and well-informed decisions, we need a clear understanding of the differences among the terms used when describing natural/bioidentical and synthetic hormones.

Synthetic/Nonhuman Identical Hormones. Whether estrogen (Premarin, ethinyl estradiol; see Chapter 9) or progestogens (Medroxyprogesterone, Provera, levonorgestrel, Norethindrone, norethindrone acetate, desogestrel, norgestimate, and so on; see

Chapter 9) are all foreign to our body because their molecular formulas are unlike any hormones human bodies make.

The reason they alleviate some of the symptoms is because our cells misread certain portions of the molecular structure of these substances. If you are currently on HRT you are possibly taking one of the nonhuman identical hormones—and may not be getting the results you need and desire.

How Nonhuman Identical Hormones Were Developed— A Little Bit of History

Insulin, the hormone that saves the lives of diabetic patients, was initially obtained from animal sources. Pork and beef insulin came to market more than 50 years ago and saved children with juvenile diabetes whose lives would have been cut short by the horrific disease.

The enormous success of insulin opened the door for the development of other animal-based hormones. However, within a short period side-effects surfaced. Kidney failure and blindness were discovered to develop in patients who used animal source insulin. The situation motivated the change to human insulin. Once human insulin arrived to the market, beef and pork insulin disappeared and the side-effects were dramatically reduced. Today, human insulin preparations save the lives of millions. They are bioidentical formulations of insulin and no one argues their superiority over insulin made from pork or beef.

Unlike insulin, estrogen for menopausal women took a different route.

Initially extracted from pregnant Canadian women's urine, the estrogen used to treat menopausal women, although human identical and perfectly matched for women, proved too expensive and the industry moved toward animal source, cheaper estrogens.

Estrogen extracted from pregnant mares' urine came into existence in the 1940s. Since then, it has remained the primary and most lucrative source of estrogens made by the major pharmaceutical companies (Wyeth-Ayerst and now Pfizer). Because its use was not very extensive at the start, little was learned and addressed about side-effects arising from the use of pregnant mares' estrogen (conjugated equine estrogen, brand name Premarin). By the 1970s, side-effects of this animal source estrogen began to surface. Premarin used without progestin increases the risk for endometrial cancer. Another hormone drug, Provera (medroxyprogesterone acetate), was created to eliminate that side-effect. By 2002 when the WHI study was discontinued, Premarin was the biggest seller in the U.S. with $2 billion projected for 2002.

Despite the findings of the WHI, Premarin was never taken off the market and continues to be widely prescribed to the tune of $500 million a year. It seems odd since clearly the insulin lesson was lost on estrogen.

Premarin contains a few humanlike estrogen molecules but it also contains equilin, equilenin, and 200 other molecules specific to the horse but foreign to women.

Questions on how equilin and equilenin affect estrogen receptors in humans abound and many studies have demonstrated the significant and nefarious difference between the actions of human identical estradiol and horse estrogens. From the way horse estrogen disturbs human DNA, to the way it increases coronary artery spasms, to how it increases bad fats in our blood, disrupts bleeding parameters, to how it negatively affects our brain, problems abound.

And just think, if there were no better option, then ok, but the option of bioidentical hormones has always been there. That makes the situation even more disturbing.

Progestin (medroxy progesterone acetate, Provera) is the synthetic progesterone created specifically in a laboratory to offset the negative side-effect of horse urine estrogen (Premarin), which has been connected to increased incidence and risk of endometrial overgrowth and cancer. Provera is also used to induce menstruation when a woman's period is late.

To even call it progesterone is to do women and the medical profession a disservice. Medroxyprogesterone acetate does not resemble natural progesterone in its actions. It is a chemical compound with a formula very loosely resembling that of progesterone.

Provera was created in the 1970s when the dangers of Premarin (conjugated equine estrogen) replacement were first published in the medical literature. Oddly, it's easier and safer to use micronized progesterone, which is human identical and proven safer in every study.

Used alone without estrogens, medroxyprogesterone acetate increases risk of blood clots and cancer.

It is critical to avoid confusing progestin with natural/bioidentical progesterone.

Progesterone is the human identical hormone our body makes to balance the action of estrogen. Progesterone is safe and necessary to our well-being. In IVF and other fertility treatments progesterone, the micronized, human identical, bioidentical hormone is used routinely in oral, injectable or intravaginal forms.

Provera (medroxyprogesterone acetate) *should never be used*.

The Latest in FDA-Approved Menopausal Therapies

In the past year two drugs received FDA approval. One is **Osphena**, a non-hormone synthetic drug recommended for the treatment of vaginal dryness and atrophy and **Brisdelle**, an antidepressant-like drug recommended for treatment of hot flashes. The drugs have been on the market less than two years, giving them no track record of safety or efficacy. Sadly, they also don't treat the root cause of the problem which is hormone loss. They only treat symptoms.

How Natural/Bioidentical Hormones Reach the Consumer Market

Natural/bioidentical/human identical hormones are sold by the manufacturer in powder form in large drums. The manufacturer sells the raw natural progesterone, estriol, estradiol, testosterone, thyroid, etc., in the powder form directly to either small pharmacies or large pharmaceutical companies. They all get the same raw material. From this point, the final product is either made individually in compounding pharmacies or in standardized large-scale pharmaceutical products for sale to pharmacies and then to the public. Both are prescription medications.

There is no difference between the active ingredients in FDA-approved or compounded hormones. The confusion is purely semantics.

FDA-approved bioidenticals are the same as compounded bioidenticals. They just come in different formulations and are manufactured under different regulatory agencies: FDA under federal while compounded under state pharmacy boards.

Prometrium is an example of the FDA-approved oral version of natural/bioidentical/micronized progesterone mixed in a peanut oil base, produced by a large pharmaceutical company and distributed by prescription, for sale at all pharmacies.

The same progesterone can be made in a specific compounded form to be made for use by individual patients, in a compounding pharmacy equipped to create custom orders in cream or injectable, intravaginal or oral forms, following your doctor's orders.

When Monica at the age of 47 started going through perimenopause she asked her gynecologist what to do. The doctor gave her Premarin and Provera and sent her on her way. Monica did not do well with that regimen. Her symptoms got worse. She had hot flashes, night sweats kept her up all night, and the brain fog made her feel loopy. She called her doctor and asked about natural/

bioidentical hormones. Her doctor said that they don't work; that they are a marketing scam drummed up by a TV actress, and that all hormone preparations are the same. He told her to stay on the hormones he prescribed.

Dissatisfied with this answer, Monica came to see me. I explained the difference. The problem is that the TV actress who promotes the bioidenticals as a new option available to women isn't doing anyone any favors. Bioidentical is a marketing term referring to human identical hormones that have been around for decades and can either be found by prescription at your local pharmacy or individually compounded at a compounding pharmacy. After about a month on human identical hormones Monica felt great, but she continued to see her gynecologist for PAP smears and regular exams yet never told him she changed hormone preparations. To this day, her doctor doesn't know she's taking natural/bioidentical hormones.

I know too many patients like Monica. The situation is tragic. It is a poor reflection on the relationship between doctor and patient and it keeps the truth and reality of natural/bioidentical hormones away from too many doctors and women who desperately need to know about them. It prevents more women from gaining access to natural/bioidentical hormones because if everyone told the truth, doctors would have no option but to learn the difference between hormones and treat women with human identicals all the time.

Why Doesn't Your Conventional Doctor Know the Difference Between Human Identical and Nonhuman Identical Hormones Still?

The reasons natural/bioidentical hormones are still not universally accepted and ignorant doctors tell you they aren't good are many:

1. After the WHI study, conventional physicians were scared and indoctrinated by the media and their medical societies to stop prescribing any kind of sex hormones.

As a result, more than 7 million women were taken off hormones. The doctors, afraid of lawsuits, still don't like prescribing hormones even though the results of the WHI study have been disproven and the need for hormones has been unquestionably proven.

2. Physicians get their information from medical journals, at medical conferences and mostly from the pharmaceutical drug representatives who visit their offices. As a result, most physicians in clinical practice only know what they were taught during training which could have been decades old and clearly outdated but surely what special interest drug companies are marketing to them.

3. Physicians are more afraid of lawsuits than caring for the patient, and the relationship between doctors and patients has been deteriorating over the past two decades. Thus physicians will avoid confrontation or any situation they may perceive as jeopardizing the status quo even if it may be in the best interest of the patient.

4. Ob/gyns should be those to prescribe hormone therapies for menopausal women. They do prescribe birth control pills in teens with impunity and work with hormones in IVF. Instead they are unlikely to know how to treat menopausal women without scaring them. A big problem is created by conventional gynecologists who are not up-to-date on the use of hormones in wellness and disease prevention and don't take the time to learn about them. Sadly, they don't tell the patient "I don't know," which is the truth. Sadly, they label the usage of bioidentical hormones as quackery and in the process deprive women from getting good preventive medical care.

5. For the past five decades gynecologists have been indoctrinated by their medical societies and by the drug representatives to prescribe birth control pills to young

women and Premarin and Provera to menopausal women. These are both nonhuman identical hormones which carry significant risks. They may cause infertility, cancer, blood clots, strokes, heart attacks, and premature death. However, doctors continue to prescribe these dangerous medications with impunity because they are following purely financially motivated groups, missing their Hippocratic mission to serve the patient's best interests.

6. Pharmaceutical representatives regularly visit doctors' offices with samples of their newest drugs. Along with the free samples, they distribute pseudo-scientific studies hailing the value of the very medications they promote. When evaluating these medications, doctors must keep in mind that the manufacturer of the product always sponsors the referenced research.

This scenario also occurs in continuing medical education courses and articles published in medical journals. An inordinately large portion of medical information reaches doctors courtesy of pharmaceutical companies. Doctors must ask themselves if the research is reputable as the study was conducted and paid for by the company that stands to financially benefit from the study's positive results. Pharmaceutical companies spend millions of dollars on marketing and publicity for their patented medications, because of the huge revenues they bring.

Natural/bioidentical hormones, although their molecular formulas are identical to human hormones that occur in nature, can get patents when using special delivery systems (gels, patches, pills—called use patent). Ironically, the same manufacturers that make Premarin and Provera in the U.S. make bioidentical progesterone in Europe. It is sad to see how Americans get the short end of the stick when studies and FDA-approved bioidentical hormones abound in other areas of the world yet inferior products are sold in the U.S.

But there is hope. A large pharmaceutical company called Besins has patents on bioidentical estradiol (Estrogel) and progesterone (Utrogestan, Progestogel) but it's a company started in Europe and now headquartered in Asia so competition with the U.S. pharmaceutical giants has kept it from seriously penetrating the market and getting the information to doctors and patients. Abbott is another big pharma who has only now broken into the U.S. market with huge marketing dollars spent on Androgel, which is human identical testosterone gel for andropausal men (low T).

Natural/Bioidentical/Human Identical Hormones Is the Solution

After many years of getting poor or no results with conventional HRT (nonhuman identical hormone replacement) in my practice, the option to offer my patients natural/bioidentical hormones came to save the day and the quality of life of thousands of women.

When Ellen came to see me, she was in her early 40s. The first time I saw her, I wasn't prescribing natural/bioidentical hormones routinely in my practice. Ellen had complaints of weight gain, change in her periods and stomach problems. A thorough examination and gastrointestinal work-up failed to make a diagnosis in Ellen. Together, we decided to try Ellen on birth control pills. Scientific or maybe mostly marketing pseudo-scientific data supporting the use of birth control pills in perimenopausal women abounded and the use of birth control pills through menopausal changes was routine in Europe at the time. After three months on birth control pills, Ellen returned to my office in tears. She felt worse. Her breasts had ballooned, her sex drive completely disappeared, the migraines had worsened and her mood was foul. She was miserable with the results and wanted something else. I decided to try natural/bioidentical hormones (they were known as natural in those days). Since there were no such products in the FDA-approved category

123

at the time, I found a compounding pharmacy that did a lot of work with hospitals and had them compound the hormones for Ellen. Two weeks after starting the natural hormones (17-beta estradiol and progesterone in cream form), miraculously, Ellen's symptoms began to vanish and she was her happy old self again.

Ellen's story was a tipping point for me. The effectiveness and superiority of natural/bioidentical hormones did not go unnoticed to me. I read all the scientific studies on natural hormones and was stunned how different than the drugs I was prescribing before they were. Their actions in the body were safe and effective, just like our own hormones when we are young and healthy.

Laura, another patient, was 16 and had severe PMS and cramps that incapacitated her every month. Her mother took her to the gynecologist, who offered one option: birth control pills. Her mother felt uncomfortable and brought Laura to me. One year earlier I would have given Laura birth control pills as well. However, the success with natural/bioidentical hormones was so impressive that I started her on natural/bioidentical progesterone for two weeks before her period. Laura felt great and had none of the negative side-effects of birth control pills (mood swings, swollen breasts, weight gain).

Over the span of a few months, I found myself—a conventional doctor who followed classical approaches to treating problems following conventional medical protocols-- suddenly switching all my patients with hormone imbalances to natural/bioidentical/ human identical hormones. The results were remarkable. I could treat each patient as an individual because I had the ability to fine-tune the amounts of hormones I used with the help of compounding pharmacies, and my patients were happy. No other treatment in my medical practice offered such satisfaction or consistent success. I searched the literature for protocols and education on the use of compounding and dosing of bioidentical hormones but came up with nothing. In time, I developed my own protocols. Ellen, Laura and hundreds of other women were our pioneers and many others followed. And to this day (20+ years later) no one I've treated has returned to nonhuman identical hormones, antidepressants, birth control pills or other treatments. And to boot, we are all still on the hormones and will stay on them because there is no scientifically sound reason to stop.

In our office we have a team member who calls patients who no longer work with us to find out why they left the practice so we can learn from them. Invariably, no one leaves because of negative side-effects, cancers or lack of kindness or support from us. I am proud to say our practice (Evolved Science- eshealth.com) is a model of "truly evolved health care," what true prevention and its practice must become if our health care system can survive and truly help people lead healthier and better quality lives.

Natural/Bioidentical/Human Identical Hormones Are Available by Prescription Only

There is a huge disconnect between what the public knows about bioidenticals and how to best benefit from their usage. Even if Oprah or other celebrities endorse them, they aren't doctors and even if they recommend doctors, they may not be recommending the right one for you. Without access to unbiased, significant, evidence-based scientific data and training on the use of natural/ bioidentical/human identical hormones in wellness and disease prevention, neither conventional nor alternative doctors are able to become knowledgeable or experienced enough to treat you successfully. Without sponsorship for more research and with a lack of conventional training programs, the scientific data and instruction on clinical use of natural/bioidentical hormones is intentionally kept away from the majority of physicians who could easily prescribe them and many of whom would gladly do it.

Confusion about terminology and special interest groups stop progress at every step of the journey. Just look at how difficult it has been for me to get here and be able to explain the difference between natural, bioidentical, human identical and synthetic, nonhuman identical hormone preparations. Terminology is intentionally confusing, and the same information is recycled for decades, stopping new information from reaching you. The result: conventionally trained doctors maintain a defensive attitude toward hormones, they don't listen to your needs, so they cannot help you. Sadly, most of them don't really care.

Few physicians take the time, do the research to find a good training program, or take on the expense to build a solid natural/bioidentical hormone practice. This situation does an enormous disservice to women who are desperately searching for help when the solution is constantly paraded right in front of them on TV and the internet.

How You Can Get Natural/Bioidentical/Human Identical Hormones

To get natural/bioidentical hormones, you need a prescription. Prescriptions can only be written by licensed professionals: physician, physician assistant, or nurse practitioner (depending on the state). The prescription is then filled at a regular pharmacy if using FDA-approved bioidentical hormones or a compounding pharmacy for a specific/individualized dose formulations (testosterone does not exist in FDA-approved formulation for women, thus has to be compounded).

How do you find a knowledgeable, experienced and caring doctor who will listen to you, figure out your needs and write the correct prescription for you? Or how do you convince your present doctor to prescribe bioidentical estradiol and progesterone instead of the nonhuman identical drugs?

Compounding

The practice of pharmacy and medicine are legislated and supervised at the individual state level. According to the New York State Board of Pharmacy, any licensed pharmacy can add *compounding* to its list of services. Each state has its own rules, but in general once licensed by the individual State Board of Pharmacy, any pharmacy can technically mix medication per doctor's orders.

Lists of compounding pharmacies specializing in filling prescriptions for natural/bioidentical hormones are easily found on search engines.

The best compounding pharmacies are those dedicated to compounding. They provide unique services and individualized care. To achieve optimum results it is imperative you find a physician who is trained and experienced in working with compounding. I cannot stress the importance of your doctor knowing and understanding the particular compounding pharmacy and its practices well.

Compounding pharmacies have been around for hundreds of years. In fact, pharmaceutical companies are outgrowths of compounding. Every medication you receive from a hospital or office (we provide extensive IV infusion services at our practice) IV bag (e.g., antibiotics, medications, vitamins, etc.) is compounded. Much of the medication compounded is made to order accounting for patient allergies, intolerance to certain formulations or just plain lack of availability of a particular dose or type of medication. Your dog and cat and pretty much most of veterinary medicine relies on compounding for much of their medications. Topical painkillers and other medications specifically made for the individual patient are also compounded. Compounding is ubiquitous to the delivery of medications. Many insurance companies reimburse for compounded products. Just ask your carrier. Also, you may be interested to know that major drug companies own compounding pharmacies.

My goal in telling you all this is to help you understand that compounding is not some recently discovered novelty, but rather is and has been an integral part of medical practice for the longest time. Most physicians rely heavily on the services of compounders to get their patients the best medications, often without even being aware of it.

Don't be afraid to ask your physician what he/she thinks and even more importantly knows about the use of natural/bioidentical hormones. He/she may already know something about them or may want to learn more. He/she may feel comfortable to write a prescription and help you get it filled. If your doctor is not receptive, change doctors. Find one who has experience with natural/bioidentical/human identical hormones on more than 200 patients and has received formal training in the area. Better Health Initiative, www.bhionline.org, is a not-for-profit organization of a group of physicians (including me) founded in 2007. It provides online education and in-office clinical training for qualified physicians who want to practice prevention and work with bioidentical hormones. Affiliated with one of the NYC medical schools our physicians receive continuing medical education credits for their training.

Today, there are more than 3,000 physicians in the U.S. and internationally trained by our team of leading physicians.

For more information please go to www.bhionline.org and we will help you find the right physician or nurse practitioner for you.

If your own physician is interested in learning, take this book to him/her and suggest they contact us at www.bhionline.org for more information and support.

CHAPTER 7

The Human Identical Hormone Program for You: Guidelines You Must Know

When I first started working with bioidentical hormones I realized there had to be many options and various formulations. After doing my research I started with transdermal preparations and stayed with them until I acquired extensive expertise at prescribing them. In addition, as the results of the WHI came tumbling in, problems with the use of oral estrogen and its toxicity to the liver reinforced my work with creams. Transdermal, preparations were easily and safely absorbed, study after study supporting these facts.

When I first started working with bioidentical hormones I asked my local compounding pharmacist, whose business consisted primarily of compounding for hospitals, veterinarians, and children with autism, if he could work with me to improve quality, safety, and predictability of absorption for the hormones I was committed to work with. Having researched the pharmaceutical literature on methods of administration of medications, I quickly discovered which creams were better absorbed and most bioavailable.

Transdermal creams contain the hormones in specific vehicles that are applied directly to the skin. We use areas of the body with good circulation and minimal amount of fat under the skin. That is because hormones love fat and if the cream is applied to an area with fat under it, the hormones will just stay in the fat cells and not help systemically. The best areas for optimal absorption are the inner wrists, forearms, upper inner arms, and shoulders. Absorption occurs rapidly when the correct concentration of hormones is placed in the correct creams. The frequency of allergic skin reaction is very low and just stopping the creams eliminates any problem they may have caused. (In more than 20,000 patients cared for in our practice, we've had to change the vehicle—what the cream ingredients besides the hormones are—due to rashes or itchy skin at the application site fewer than 10 times in 20-plus years.) Absorption through the skin bypasses the liver, providing less stress to the liver. While oral estradiol is also safe, it has lower absorbability than creams, requiring larger doses to reach the same blood levels.

Methods of Natural/Bioidentical Hormone Administration

The ability to offer you totally individualized therapy with human identical/bioidentical hormones depends on your physician's experience, knowledge of the therapy, care for you and good and consistent follow-up. Keep in mind we are only referring to compounded bioidentical hormones at this point. Soon we will introduce FDA-approved options and how you can use the best of both worlds in your particular case.

I find many doctors I speak to in a quandary. They want to help their patients but they are afraid. Malpractice suits, lack of support from the medical societies and lack of information have left the medical profession in shambles when it comes to this area of medicine. Nonhuman identical hormone replacement is the only form of hormones mass marketed. Doctors are aware that patients are afraid to use Premarin, Provera, even birth control pills because of side-effects and the risk of cancer, blood clots, heart attacks and strokes. But most doctors lack information on natural/bioidentical hormones they need to prescribe them with confidence. So many doctors just hedge their bets and still believe the totally debunked fact that all hormones are the same. They will tell you natural/bioidentical hormones do not work, not enough scientific studies exist, when in fact all they need is the information on how to use bioidentical hormones in their clinical practice. And with the new non-hormone drugs available to treat symptoms of menopause (Osphena and Brisdelle), there is even less help for the overwhelmed gynecologist. So I encourage you to take this book to your doctor, and any other information on natural/bioidentical hormones written by physicians with solid and extensive track record, and begin a discussion on natural/bioidentical hormone supplementation.

FDA-approved bioidentical hormone preparations do exist and there are many options you should be aware of:

- **Estradiol tablets:** 1 mg
- **Estrogel .06%** (gel form—Pump one unit dose per pump
- **Elestrin** (gel form)—Pump one unit dose per pump
- **Divigel**—Packets with gel in various doses
- **Vivelle-Dot**—Patches in various doses
- **Minivelle**—Patches in various doses
- **Climara**—Patches in various doses
- **Estrace**—Tablets in various doses
- **Estradiol**—Tablets in various doses
- **Prometrium**—Peanut oil caps in various doses
- **Progesterone**—Capsules and tablets in various doses

The Hormone Supplementation Program

My two decades of experience has shown that most people easily fit into one of the five groups we've been discussing based on age and symptoms.

Before you decide that natural/bioidentical hormones are what you need, you should try to identify into which group you may fit. Undergoing a thorough evaluation by your physician, discussing your symptoms and your history will ensure proper and successful identification of the best treatment options for you. The internet isn't going to really help you.

- ▶ Low doses of progesterone in the younger group for two weeks before periods is an easy and safe way to start.
- ▶ As you move into the more advanced groups adding estradiol for up to 10 days in the middle of the month and progesterone the last two weeks of the month are easy ways to provide balance.
- ▶ As we enter the menopausal groups continuous administration of both estradiol and progesterone works best to help eliminate most symptoms.
- ▶ During postmenopause, decreasing progesterone to one week a month and keeping estradiol for the entire month consistently works in our patient population.
- ▶ Taking breaks every few months if no menses are present is a good way to detoxify the system.

A well-trained and experienced physician will help you find the ideal balance for your needs.

If your physician is interested in learning our protocols please recommend they go to www.bhionline.org.

Statistics

When researching scientific studies on hormone replacement therapies, conventional research offers a wide array of confusing and contradictory information. Most findings published in the highly respected U.S. Pub Med literature resource database lists academic studies on hormone replacement with nonhuman identical hormones (those that were proven to increase risk of heart attacks, stroke and cancer in the WHI study) with little or no distinction made among different types of hormones and their action in the human body.

When you read results of scientific data or listen to media reports, you are immediately hit by numbers—statistics. The world of statistics focuses on collecting data from large groups of people from various cohorts (e.g., young, old, college-educated, married, single, living in houses, with high blood pressure, with allergies, and so on), searching common denominators, then applying the data to you as an individual. Some data assure us that estrogen protects us from heart disease and osteoporosis, while other data contradict. The biggest problem is that statistics **do not apply to the individual**. Statistics refer to populations and are then manipulated by special interest to fit desired results to prompt you to buy specific medication, undergo certain procedures, take certain immunizations and buy specific clothes, technology, cars, watch certain TV shows, and so forth. Statistics are used by marketers to sell. In medicine, they are consistently used to scare or bully you into complying with the special interest group that spends the most money on marketing its products/technology and so on.

When it comes to hormone therapies we are faced with the same dilemma.

To the public and doctors the data is confusing because we have been indoctrinated to believe that all hormone preparations are the same. When deciding what type of hormone treatment you choose, I caution you against relying on statistics and data presented by the bias of special interest groups. Don't let statistics bully you into a particular course of action. **It's your life and you are the only statistic of 100 percent.**

Thyroid Supplementation

Thyroid supplementation is equally as important as estradiol, progesterone, and testosterone since once you supplement sex hormones, thyroid deficiencies become even more obvious.

Determining thyroid function through blood tests is essentially useless. TSH levels in the blood has been considered the gold standard for the diagnosis of hypothyroidism for more than five decades. It is outdated and useless if we are looking to prevent disease and treat people rather than numbers on paper. Using the results of the TSH test to make treatment decisions creates more problems than it solves. When patients are treated with thyroid medication, TSH levels drop significantly and doctors react by telling the patient they are hyperthyroid when in fact they are normal. Physicians also scare the patient who takes thyroid medication into believing the medication will negatively affect their heart and bones, which is scientifically unfounded.

Using noninvasive diagnostic tools for the diagnosis of (euthyroid sick syndrome) hypothyroidism in prevention, before patients become seriously ill, is more logical, simpler, safe, and prevents illness.

Below is the common-sense evidence based approach to diagnosing low thyroid in prevention:

- ▶ Morning basal body temperature (never reaches normal 98.6°)
- ▶ Basal metabolic rate (always low)
- ▶ Bloating
- ▶ Dry, itchy skin
- ▶ Foggy thinking
- ▶ Fatigue
- ▶ Weight gain or inability to lose weight in spite of adequate effort, and so forth

▶ Water retention
▶ Sleep disturbances
▶ Loss of libido
▶ Cold intolerance
▶ Depression
▶ Constipation
▶ Hair loss
▶ Loss of eyebrow hair and definition
▶ Palpitations (mostly at night and at rest)

All symptoms in the preceding list are objective and subjective findings that represent the most important factor, the patient.

Symptoms correctly interpreted by a knowledgeable physician who isn't limited in his/her thinking by outdated rules or fear will confirm the diagnosis of low thyroid regardless of what your endocrinologist tells you about the results of your blood test. Cold intolerance, weight gain, loss of libido, foggy thinking, bloating, hot flashes and night sweats, constipation, hair loss and loss of eyebrow hair, coarse, dry, itchy skin, and palpitations are all symptoms of thyroid deficiency that rarely correlate to the results of outdated blood testing.

In our practice, when a patient comes in with these complaints we will start a low dose of a combination of thyroid hormones (T3 and T4). The treatment has *never* made any patient hyperthyroid in more than two decades of clinical experience. Thyroid hormone supplementation when correctly diagnosed and safely treated increases energy production. Both men and women consistently feel better without increasing the risk of heart disease or osteoporosis. We have never used thyroid supplementation as a tool for weight loss. The average follow-up for our patients is 5 to 10 years.

The duration of treatment is dictated by the individual patient need and the advice of a knowledgeable, open-minded and caring doctor whose job is to serve the patient, not follow blindly outdated rules stating that treatment be based solely on TSH results.

Use the preceding guidelines to work with your doctor in developing the therapeutic program that works best for you. Do not try to do it yourself or work with a provider who isn't experienced.

Prevention represents health and wellness, which are the sum total of diet, exercise, supplements, sleep, stress management, hormones, and many other variables that must be taken into consideration.

Medical subspecialists don't have the correct tools to help you stay healthy and live a high-quality life. They only look to find diseases and place labels in their limited area of expertise without taking into consideration the infinite number of variables that affect overall outcome. Breaking the human body down into organ systems and even smaller parts only serves to create a dangerous and disjointed picture. Find one doctor to be your partner to understand you and oversee and coordinate your entire care and use subspecialists for specific needs only.

Long-Term Use of Natural/Bioidentical Hormone Supplementation

In the resource section of the book, you will find references to studies on the effects of natural/bioidentical hormone supplementation. Because my goal is to bring doctors and patients together on the topic of natural/bioidentical hormones I've listed scientific references at the end of this book for you to take to your doctor and start an intelligent conversation about bioidentical hormones. Have your doctors read the studies. They are all from reputable mainstream scientific publications.

CHAPTER 8

Clearing Up the Confusion About Medical Testing

In our culture, medical testing is perceived as symbolic of good medical care. Various opinions on what constitutes adequate testing abound in medical journals, training programs, and lay sources of information (Google, social media, pop literature, women's journals, TV shows and news, and newspapers). Daily, I am faced with the same questions, from new patients and physicians: "What tests will you use to determine what hormone regimen to design for me specifically? How will you protect me against potential dangers and how will you measure the effectiveness of treatment? What are the results of my blood tests?"

To properly answer these questions, we must fully appreciate that blood testing straddles two worlds.

1. The first is the world of conventional medicine, where all testing is geared towards diagnosing disease. This world includes what is often incorrectly labeled as preventive medicine, a branch of conventional medicine, aimed at early diagnosis of disease, but not really disease

prevention (mammograms, PSA, colonoscopy, Pap smears, and so on).

2. The second is the world of wellness where true prevention exists. Our world is caught between conventional medicine and alternative practices. Most people live most of their lives in wellness. Illnesses represent minor interruptions in a continuum of health. More than 95% of the world population never see a doctor. In the world of wellness and true prevention everyone has one common goal: to prolong and optimize the healthy periods and shorten or even prevent illnesses (acute and chronic).

Natural/bioidentical/human identical hormone therapies belong in the world of true prevention.

True prevention is an emerging field in health care. Medical information gathered about our genetic make-up (telomeres, stem cells, DNA, genetic markers, gene mapping), environmental impact and lifestyles (diet, exercise, stress management), supplements, hormones and other modalities (acupuncture, meditation, aromatherapy, energy healing, naturopathy, and so forth) are used in concert to improve our odds of living a longer, healthier, high-quality life.

Wellness and true prevention is about helping women and men (Chapter 9) feel better, improve quality of and enjoy life, ultimately preventing disease.

The easiest way to measure success in this newly developing medical field of true prevention is to identify symptoms early and treat their root cause swiftly and safely. While symptom relief is the goal, it isn't like treating a headache with Tylenol. It is about understanding what causes the headache (low estrogen, neck out of balance, dietary indiscretions, sedentary lifestyle, and so forth) and then treating the causes.

For instance, a hangover may cause a bad headache. In order to properly solve the problem, you have to make the connection between drinking too much alcohol and the headache and then, following the "best practice" approach, treat it with lots of nonalcoholic fluids, IV infusions, and rest. Also, the *main* lesson is to decrease the amount of alcohol you drink the next time to **prevent** the hangover and headache from occurring altogether. This approach accomplishes two goals:

1. Increases self-awareness and helps you make important connections in your own body.
2. Prevents you from worsening the original problem (e.g., taking NSAIDs that cause gastric irritation, getting more dehydrated—resulting in more medical problems).

No medical test can give you this crucial information.
Because true prevention is a new field in conventional medicine and I am a conventional physician, my experience and clinical practice have taught me and our team to integrate blood testing into our patient care, modifying and focusing its use on wellness and disease prevention.

1. We test your bloods initially to have a baseline for your hormone levels and general blood picture, at a time when presumably your symptoms were the worst.
2. Once we worked together for a few months and optimized your hormone balance, diet, exercise and other parameters, we repeat the bloods so we have a measurement of your hormone levels and general blood picture when you are feeling your best.

The following list of tests is currently recommended as part of our routine medical maintenance programs. They may represent our standard but we never forget each one of us is an individual and the decision to have a test or a treatment is ultimately yours.

Pap Smear

Your gynecologist will encourage you to have annual or even biannual Pap smears. The test was developed to diagnose early cervical abnormalities that are easily, safely and successfully treated as well as HPV infections that may lead to problems later on. Statistically, the standard profile for women at high risk for getting cervical cancer include young women in their teens and 20s, of less affluent background, with multiple sexual partners. Cervical cancer is also a disease caused by few of the hundreds of HPV viruses more than 90 percent of sexually active people are infected with over the course of their lives. The people at risk are women who do not get regular check-ups. Those who do will be at lowest risk and treatment is curative.

If you do not belong in the above cohort, your chances of getting cervical cancer are negligible and the need for frequent Pap tests becomes questionable. In fact, in the early 2000s, the Preventive Medicine Task Force of the National Institutes of Health recommended that women with two consecutive normal Pap smears a year apart do not need Pap smears on a yearly basis. I would also like to add that older women, over 50 with limited sexual activity and exposure to one partner who is monogamous, may not need Pap smears more than once every five years.

Confer with your gynecologist about the frequency of Pap smears indicated for your particular situation. Make sure the doctor notices you and addresses your particular situation. Keep in mind that the results of the Pap smear do not indicate the effectiveness or impact of hormone therapy. Also keep in mind your gynecologist is trained to do regular Pap smears and gets paid for doing them. Hence, the incentive is to do Pap smears. Ask why you need the test and what the appropriate frequency is. Ask what the doctor will do with the results of the test? How will results affect therapeutic course?

Blood Tests

At Kings County Hospital in Brooklyn, New York, where I received my training, we routinely removed more than 100cc of blood from every patient admitted to the hospital in constant search for abnormal results. Students, interns, residents, fellows, all products of the U.S. medical school training, aren't allowed to question protocols and must follow blindly the system of indoctrination. Four decades later with experience gained from thousands of patients, I can unequivocally tell you two things:

▶ Test results don't necessarily reflect what's going on with a patient.

▶ Only perform tests whose results will substantively affect treatment.

General Blood Testing

▶ CBC (Complete blood count)—This test will diagnose anemia and the distribution and details about red and white blood cells. This test is important in menstruating women because they are frequently anemic from blood loss and a diet low in iron. It's also important for men who take testosterone, which increases red blood cell count.

▶ General/comprehensive/metabolic profile—This is an evaluation of liver and kidney functions, hydration status, levels of calcium, magnesium, sodium, potassium, bicarbonate and other elements. Minor abnormalities are usually insignificant and must fit into the clinical picture.

▶ Lipid profile—A complete cholesterol count and its breakdown into good and bad cholesterol, triglycerides, HDL, LDL, VLDL, size of lipid particles, all with the goal of looking for the risk of heart disease. Estrogen and thyroid depletion are associated with a rise in cholesterol as well as an increase in bad cholesterol (LDL). Before considering taking a statin drug with its numerous negative side-effects, make sure your hormones are in balance. With proper hormone balance, diet and exercise as well as supplements, you will minimize the risk of heart disease over time. Study after study finds that diet and exercise are the best tools in preventing heart disease. In my experience, hormone balance is a crucial and overlooked part of the cholesterol picture. In our practice, patients have normal cholesterol values without the use of statins.

▶ Thyroid panel (TSH, free T3, free T4, TBG, TPO)— These are tests used for the past 50 years to evaluate thyroid function, used to diagnose diseases like viral and autoimmune thyroiditis (Hashimoto), and so on. Thyroid function, just like sex hormone function, decreases with age. Low thyroid is of epidemic proportion in the U.S. due to multiple factors, including environmental toxins, food preservatives, hormone therapies with birth control pills, and other medications that negatively affect and suppress normal hormone production. The blood tests mentioned above do not reliably tell the real thyroid story. Because the tests were developed to diagnose disease, the results only confuse the doctors who don't have the knowledge or training to interpret them correctly from the perspective of prevention. As a result, many patients are intimidated and scared by doctors into believing thyroid supplementation may be harmful instead of protective based solely on blood test irregularities, which prove inconsequential to the clinical picture in the long run.

Blood Testing for Hormones

Increasing numbers of experts agree that following blood hormone levels when a patient is healthy is useful beyond baseline. In our practice, we follow hormone levels with two important goals: To see what they look like when you're in ideal balance (when you feel your best) and when you are out of balance.

The following are the most commonly used tests to determine hormone status:

▶ **FSH** (Follicle-stimulating hormone)—The hormone found in humans and other mammals. Synthesized and secreted by cells called gonadotropes in the anterior pituitary gland, FSH regulates the development, growth, pubertal maturation, and reproductive processes of the body. FSH and luteinizing hormone, also produced by the pituitary gland (LH), act synergistically (in concert) in reproduction. Specifically, an increase in FSH secretion by the anterior pituitary causes ovulation. An elevated FSH number tells us the ovaries and adrenals are not making enough estrogen and progesterone to maintain fertility. The pituitary gland (and hypothalamus) sends pulses of hormones to the ovaries and adrenals, telling the ovary to ripen and release a follicle (egg) to make more estrogen, progesterone and testosterone to sustain the egg and possibly a pregnancy. FSH levels measured on Day 2 of the menstrual cycle are used to determine fertility status. If the FSH levels are low, below 10 or even 5 ng/dl, the woman is considered fertile. Women in menopause have FSH levels above 20ng/dl. It is important to note that women will have fluctuating levels of FSH over the course of the month and that is also true for menopausal women. Taking any type of hormone preparations will affect FSH levels. Persistently high FSH numbers in a young woman may be a sign of premature ovarian failure. This can be caused by ovarian suppression from medications, as a consequence of IVF, cancer treatments or other hormonal manipulation. Birth control pills suppress normal hormone production, leaving users with menopausal hormone levels.

▶ **LH** (Luteinizing hormone—Also known as lutropin and sometimes lutrophin, this is a hormone produced by gonadotrope cells in the anterior pituitary gland. An acute rise of LH triggers ovulation and growth of the corpus luteum. In males, LH is known as interstitial cell-stimulating hormone (ICSH), inducing Leydig cell production of testosterone in the testicles. LH acts synergistically with FSH. It is unnecessary for the management of hormone supplementation in older women who are menopausal. It is used in fertility work as a marker for ovulation. Another potential use of LH level is to correlate it with night sweats. An interesting theory for the source of night sweats is that the pituitary gland sends pulses of LH in the middle of the night in an attempt to stimulate end organs—i.e., adrenals and ovaries—to make more estrogen and progesterone. As these hormones become depleted by our 40s the LH and FSH pulses from the pituitary (and hypothalamus) are often futile attempts to revive the unresponsive end-organs, leading to more hot flashes and night sweats.

▶ **Estrogen** (Estradiol, Estriol, Estrone)—This is a steroid hormone made of three known components with varying degrees of activity. When we perform the tests to measure how much estrogen is in our bloodstream, we only measure the amounts of estrogen circulating freely in the bloodstream. Most estrogen is actually tied to other molecules (SHBG, or sex hormone binding globulin) and receptors on the cell walls, and cannot be measured by our present methods of testing. It is useful to know how much of the hormone supplementation taken by a patient gets into the bloodstream. It helps determine the reliability of the formulation of hormones used—creams vs. pills vs. patches. By measuring the amount of hormone in the blood, we find out how well it gets absorbed, and by listening to the patient we know how the hormone affects them in real life. That combination of information leads to truly remarkable and useful results.

▶ **Estradiol,** is the most effective estrogen used in hormone supplementation. A level around 50 ng/dl may be most protective and if the patient feels well, balance is achieved. Things become a bit complicated when the estradiol level is high or low and the patient still feels well. If the level is high (> 200), we repeat the test to eliminate the possibility of lab error or that the patient may have applied the estradiol cream close in time or location to where the blood was drawn from.

▶ **Estrone** is the estrogen of menopause and also is high in women on birth control pills. Some data seems to indicate its role isn't dangerous but its use is unclear.

▶ **Estriol** is the estrogen of pregnancy and its use in nonpregnant or menopausal women is limited. In our practice, we use it to help improve vaginal lining and as a face cream. It can only be obtained by prescription from a compounding pharmacy. You need a knowledgeable physician to order the proper dosage and delivery vehicle. Since estradiol is well studied and delivers excellent results there is no good reason to use either estriol or estrone in hormone supplementation.

▶ **Progesterone**—Measuring free progesterone levels is of no use unless the patient is receiving progesterone supplementation. Alternative practitioners recommend a progesterone to estrogen ratio of 1:10. Progesterone is used in fertility treatments. It helps support implantation of the fertilized egg into the uterus and its growth. The most bioavailable formulations in decreasing order are: injectable, intravaginal, oral and transdermal. (NB-only bioidentical/human identical/micronized progesterone is used in fertility treatments, not nonhuman identical progestins like medroxyprogesterone acetate—Provera or progestins used in birth control pills).

▶ **Testosterone**—This is a steroid sex hormone belonging to the androgen group, secreted primarily by the testicles in males and ovaries in females. Small amounts are also secreted by the adrenal glands. On average, in adult males, the plasma concentration of testosterone is about 7 to 8 times the levels in adult females, but as the metabolic consumption of testosterone in males is much greater, the daily production is about 20 times greater in men. Information on normal testosterone values in women doesn't exist and a lack of studies to correlate testosterone levels to symptoms leaves us in a position where we learn with each new patient. Testosterone levels appear higher in girls and women with polycystic ovarian syndrome (**PCOS**) but the medical community doesn't know the significance of this finding. Fertility research recommends the use of DHEA, a testosterone precursor, in large doses (25–50 mg three times a day) to help women get pregnant. The results of this approach are excellent and seem to negate the belief that high testosterone levels may be undesirable in women. In fact, some studies even suggest that high testosterone levels in women with PCOS may be Mother Nature's way of protecting fertility into older years because women with PCOS have a higher chance of getting pregnant as they get older. Women on birth control pills also tend to have higher testosterone levels. More about the role of testosterone in women will eventually emerge. Meanwhile we measure baseline levels when seeing a patient for the first time and follow changes over time. How the patient feels is the most important factor in deciding how to proceed with hormone therapy in prevention.

Testosterone Testing in Men

In men, there is a clearer correlation between blood testosterone levels and how the patient feels. Testing baseline and then repeating every 3–6 months during therapy provides a good perspective on levels and correlating them to patient well-being. Total testosterone levels are misleading because testosterone is tightly bound to a protein in the blood (SHBG, or sex hormone binding globulin). Free testosterone is a more reliable measurement of the amount of testosterone available to the cells. Metabolites of testosterone are important because dihydrotestosterone (DHT) is associated with hair loss, increased levels of estrogen, which may cause breast enlargement, increased abdominal girth, and shrinking testicles. Low estrogen levels aren't good either. A recent study has shown that men with low estrogen levels are at higher risk of heart disease and depression, thus reinforcing the very important concept that balance between estrogen and testosterone is crucial regardless of gender.

Important Fact About Blood Tests and Their Interpretation

Each of the preceding tests reflects the level of a given hormone at the moment in time it is measured. The human body is a beautiful and dynamic system. A blood test only reflects a snapshot and will never reflect the entire moving picture.

Blood tests should not be the only determinant of the decision to treat. They are part of the bigger picture and their use should always be limited to that position.

Saliva Testing

This test claims to determine free hormone levels in the saliva. It is performed by mail order laboratories without the need for a prescription from a physician and the data on the usefulness of this test is largely anecdotal and devoid of credibility or valid clinical correlation.

While the test is cheap, noninvasive and can be made available to practically anyone, the results are useless.

The only proven use for saliva testing is in the three- or four-point cortisol testing which measures cortisol levels in the saliva at different times during the day. Some endocrinologists and wellness experts do use this test when working with adrenal function.

24-Hour Urine Testing

The 24-hour urine hormone test offers information on the metabolic breakdown of hormones. Unlike the snapshot bird's-eye view provided by blood testing, 24-hour urine testing does reflect how hormones are broken down and then excreted through our kidneys over the course of one day. The test does help find out metabolites that may increase the risk for cancer. However, it is not approved in certain states, is cumbersome because the patient has to collect every drop of urine for 24 hours and it is expensive. It may, however, help determine increased risk from treatment with estrogen and thus affect the decision to treat.

Sadly, education is not available in conventional medical training and endocrinologists have no knowledge of how to interpret the results.

Bone Density

Bone density studies may be used as baseline before treatment with hormones is begun and at yearly intervals to monitor progress.

A baseline bone density test for women in perimenopause as well as men at risk provides information about the thickness of bones at a critical point when estrogen in women and testosterone in men, hormones that protect bones, start to wane. There are quite a number of bone density tests and it is important to know how reliable they are and what type of information they give you.

The most popular is the standardized DEXA scan which compares the thickness of your hip, femur or forearm and spine to what is considered normal for your age group and body configuration in large populations (remember statistics).

Following bone density levels yearly in women at risk who are taking hormones or medications to improve bone density is a good idea.

A word of caution—Bone density testing came into fashion when a drug to treat osteoporosis came to market. The drug was specifically created for the treatment of thinning bones. Fosamax received FDA approval in 1996 and to date no scientific study has been able to prove its ability to increase bone density or prevent fractures. Yet, an entire industry has been created around osteoporosis. A condition called **osteopenia** was invented, considered to be a precursor to osteoporosis. That also led to more sales and marketing of a new class of drugs called bisphosphonates, which include alendronate (Fosamax), ibandronate (Boniva) and risedronate (Actonel). A moderately rare disease found primarily in older women, osteoporosis was previously diagnosed at autopsy. Now fear of osteoporosis and doctors overanxious to prescribe send many women to take these drugs all too often. These drugs have severe side-effects ranging from abdominal and muscle pains to shattering fractures of long bones like the femur and jaw.

Diet, muscle and strength-building exercises, supplementation with vitamin D, calcium, magnesium, and natural/bioidentical hormones supplementation are benign and safer to protect from osteoporosis and even osteopenia.

Cardiac Testing

Women over the age of 40 depleted of hormones rapidly catch up with men in incidence of heart disease. Women over 50 have the same incidence of heart disease as men and the problems increase with age. Heart disease is the number one killer of women. In the U.S. alone, more than 350,000 women die every year of heart disease.

Yet in spite of much publicity and extensive research, the medical profession and the public at large seem blissfully unaware of the impact of heart disease in women as a public health issue.

Heart attacks in women do not present with the same symptoms as in men. Women present with cough, heartburn, nausea, fatigue, and vomiting. Men present with crushing chest and jaw pain. It is important to know what your risk for heart disease is and take all the steps available to prevent it.

Regular EKGs do not predict risk of heart attacks. They show the electrical rhythm in the heart at the time of the test and electrical conduction abnormalities and past heart attacks.

Stress testing is a much better way to determine heart health.

CIMT (carotid intima-media thickness) is a noninvasive ultrasound test that shows the amount of plaque deposition in the arteries and is an excellent predictor of cardiac risk before symptoms appear. CIMT was the diagnostic test used in the Kronos Early Estrogen Prevention Study (KEEPS) that compared low-dose nonhuman identical estrogens to low-dose human identical estrogens and progesterone.

Another commonly used test is the nuclear Sestamibi—a treadmill test where the patient receives a radioactive injection that helps visualize the blood vessels (coronary arteries) of the heart. The test is safe and quite reliable and has been in use for testing men for more than 30 years. A positive or abnormal test is usually followed by an angiography, also known as a coronary arteriography.

The angiogram is an invasive test. If abnormal, it becomes a therapeutic intervention and an angioplasty—cleaning out the clogged blood vessels, placement of stents (little tubes to keep the arteries open)—is performed at the same time.

Another useful screening test demonstrating the amount of calcium deposition in the coronary arteries is the ultrafast CT scan, EBCT. A noninvasive test, this very fast CT scan highlights areas of calcification (deposition of calcium) in the coronary arteries. While reliable, it is expensive and also exposes the patient to high doses of radiation.

When having these tests, it is very important to note that different equipment (no matter how standardized) may show different results. This means you must use the same equipment over time to get truly reliable results. Also of importance is the operator in ultrasound tests. Operators change and that affects results no matter what you are told.

In our medical offices of Evolved Science in New York, www. eshealth.com ,we also use another important test: vascular reactivity. Vascular reactivity is the early predictor of risk for heart attacks and strokes. It is a noninvasive test which measures how quickly blood vessels react when blood supply is temporarily diminished by the inflation of blood pressure cuffs placed on the arms. The quicker the blood vessels react, the healthier, more flexible, and less stiff they are.

Mammography

Mammography is a radiologic test used to diagnose breast abnormalities. It is not a preventive test. Mammography diagnoses breast cancer once it is there and large enough to be seen by X-ray. Mammography does not protect from breast cancer, and it does not prevent breast cancer from growing. You know how we all dread the weeks and months before our annual mammograms, intimidated into having them by our physicians and women's groups for fear of missing a cancer. The more indoctrinated we are about the importance of yearly mammograms, the more stressed out and fearful we become about breast cancer. And stress alone is the biggest killer.

The tissue that makes up our breasts is the most radiosensitive type of tissue in the body. Every time we have a mammogram we are exposing it to radiation, which does cause cancer. If you ask the radiologists, you're told not to worry, the dosage of radiation is very low. However, research over the past four decades has raised many questions about the increased risk of breast cancer associated with mammograms. Whether about their frequency, the use of old machines producing high levels of radiation or the inevitable next step which is a biopsy, fact is, women shouldn't proceed with mammograms thinking there is no downside to them. As a doctor who hasn't forgotten the Hippocratic Oath, I feel very uncomfortable that with each passing year I see my patients getting more mammograms without being told of their dangers to the breasts we are trying to protect.

Are we really doing no harm with the millions of mammograms we perform?

When I have this conversation with my patients, we quickly discover that we are all confused. We don't want to overlook potential danger, but we also don't want to stimulate cancer growth by exposure to radiation or set in motion a path leading to more damage.

With the understanding that 30,000 women out of more than 150 million in the U.S. die of breast cancer and side-effects of its therapy yearly, my patients and I reached a significant level of comfort with the following process.

1. Baseline mammogram in all my patients by age 50 (U.S. Preventive Task Force recommendation).

2. I teach patients self-examination as a most important method of early detection.

3. Mammograms every 1 to 3 years based on family history, environmental risk factors (diets high in animal fat, dairy, alcohol, and sugar), sedentary lifestyle, smoking, stressful work hours, frequent travel, and medications (Premarin, tamoxifen, birth control pills).

4. When I find myself having difficulty helping patients make a decision (often because they are being pushed by other physicians, family, internet, and friends) I recommend the following:

   a. Breast ultrasound to help distinguish between solid and hollow masses in the breast.

   b. MRI because it is excellent at defining masses.

   c. When I reach the point where no other doctor (meaning radiologist) will help commit, I recommend stereotactic biopsies (performed under X-ray guidance). Biopsies are not benign and too many doctors are glib about recommending them. Most of the time it's to protect from malpractice suits and follow standardized public health protocols rather than help the patient.

Multiple breast biopsies increase the risk for breast cancer. So, please be careful and think twice before attacking your body and changing its natural defenses and anatomy. Aspiration where a doctor just sticks a needle blindly into a mass in your breast is dangerous and should not be done under any circumstances. Just say *No* and walk out. Don't let fear control your decisions. They are your breasts after all.

"Our Feel-Good War on Breast Cancer" by Peggy Orenstein in *The New York Times Magazine* in April 2013 is an excellent article that explains why awareness isn't saving lives. Written by a journalist with breast cancer whose sole agenda is to inform, it is a most important article, a must read. It will give you more insight into the reality of breast cancer than all the medical mumbo jumbo elsewhere.

Pelvic Ultrasound: The Best Test to Follow Impact of Hormone Treatment on the Uterus and Ovaries

Every woman on any type of HRT should have a pelvic ultrasound yearly. The pelvic ultrasound is inexpensive, noninvasive, and painless and it accurately measures the thickness of the lining of your uterus as well as the state of your ovaries. This method of follow-up is important because hormone supplementation directly affects uterus and ovaries. With aging, the uterus and ovaries should shrink but with the new generation of women indefinitely on hormone therapies that is no longer the case, so ultrasound is a great surveillance tool.

Ovarian Cysts and the Use of Ultrasound

When a 22-year-old goes to a doctor with pain in her lower abdomen on the left side (on the right it could be appendix), the doctor immediately thinks: ovarian cyst. There are more ultra-sounds of the pelvis performed on young women with bellyaches than probably any other test. We are on high alert for ovarian cysts in our 20s, then forget about them as we age. Ovarian cysts are not necessarily abnormal. They are common and their presence is not necessarily a warning sign of potential disease, or an indication for surgical intervention.

In Appendix A, we discuss the corpus luteum. When we ovulate, the egg is pushed out of the ovary and the corpus luteum replaces the space the egg occupied in the ovary. On the ovary, where the egg was pushed out, a cyst sometimes develops. The cyst may be hollow, or filled with fluid or tissue, and it grows or shrinks under the influence of circulating hormones and our genetics. Occasionally, it becomes large enough to cause discomfort. Sometimes it ruptures and causes severe pain. Even under circumstances where it does rupture, while it is painful, left alone, it resolves naturally without intervention. The pain is caused by a drop of blood released into the abdominal cavity when the cyst ruptures. The blood irritates the abdominal cavity, causing the pain. Once the blood is absorbed into the system the pain resolves. Rarely the cyst is complex: e.g., dermoid with fat, hair, teeth, and nails or twists on itself causing tremendous pain, in which case it does require surgical intervention. When taking birth control pills, the ovary is stopped from ovulating and will sometimes form cysts. Ultrasound is the best method of following the cysts and surgery is rarely necessary.

Polycystic Ovaries (PCOS)

Polycystic ovarian syndrome, aka PCOS, has become a diagnosis "du jour," meaning that any time a teen or young woman goes to the doctor with weight gain, irregular periods, hair growth on face or body, and acne, bloods are drawn, and if the testosterone level is elevated or even borderline, a pelvic ultrasound is performed. Even if the ultrasound doesn't show multiple ovarian cysts, the diagnosis of Polycystic ovarian syndrome is often made. The girl is then placed on a combination of birth control pills and metformin (Glucophage, a diabetes medication) and is often told by the doctor that she will probably be infertile. This is tragic and cruel statement for anyone to hear, most of all a young girl. It also isn't always true.

Melanie was 15 when her mother brought her to see me. She was a lovely young girl who excelled in schoolwork but who was not popular. She got her period once when she was 12 and never again. Melanie gained 30 pounds in the two years prior to seeing me in spite of rigorous exercise and a rigidly low-fat and low-sugar diet.

For some unknown reason, she kept on getting heavier with each passing year. Numerous physicians had seen Melanie. Her pediatrician recommended she see a gynecologist. Though not sexually active, Melanie and her mother went to the gynecologist, who tested her bloods and performed a pelvic ultrasound. The results were inconclusive. The doctor said they were "suggestive" of polycystic ovaries and recommended Melanie start taking birth control pills and metformin and return in six months to repeat the tests.

Panic-stricken, both Melanie and her mother scoured the internet for information on the dreaded disease the young girl had been labeled with. The internet was filled with horror stories of infertility associated with PCOS, liver problems from the metformin, and recommendations for permanent hair removal from body and face. Distressed by the research findings and the lack of connection she felt with the doctors, Melanie's mother decided to look for more benign and kinder options. They came to see me. Since my first goal is to empower patients and not scare them, I addressed the high probability that Melanie might outgrow the entire situation and the diagnosis need not follow her for the rest of her life.

This was a good starting point. I watched Melanie and her mother relax. After an extensive consultation, blood work, examination, and thoughtful evaluation of all the information, it became clear to me the primary focus should be on Melanie's thyroid. The unexplained weight gain, low basal metabolic rate, dry skin, bloated appearance, loss of hair and eyebrows, and low basal temperature all pointed to the clinical diagnosis of low thyroid. In addition, since Melanie wasn't ovulating, she wasn't making progesterone. I started by prescribing thyroid and progesterone. Within a couple of weeks Melanie started to feel better. I also added metformin to her regimen as per PCOs conventional protocols and watched Melanie completely change. A less restrictive and more gentle diet worked well too.

Melanie started losing weight and was now able to go out for a slice of pizza with her friends and her social life quickly improved, helping her feel less anxious and isolated. Then we figured out the best way for her to get much needed exercise without overwhelming her. She started getting involved in walking the family dog on local hiking trails in her neighborhood and joined the JV volleyball team at school. She also started swimming. The better she felt, the more engaged she became in her school and personal life. Five years later, Melanie has regular periods, lost 20 pounds, no longer suffers with acne, is doing well in school, and has made lots of new friends. She no longer feels the heavy burden of a label— PCOS—hanging over her head like a life sentence. This is a true success story.

In late 2013, I was invited to give a talk about PCOS at a medical conference. My presentation focused on the latest scientific studies the various genetic types and variants, lots of labels, and medical information. I also added the importance of the personal touch to the patient care and how without it all we are doing is ruining many a young woman's life. After the talk, many physicians shared their own patients' stories and their clear realization of how the combination of science and care are truly the only viable solutions.

CT, PET, and MRI

If the ultrasound of the breasts or other organs isn't helpful enough the next step is to get a CT, MRI, or PET scan. These are advanced tests and should not be used routinely. Conventional medicine has infinite numbers of protocols for diagnosing illness that include extensive testing. These tests are overused in acute medicine settings and don't belong in true prevention. Oddly, every patient I see who lands in the ER for any kind of abdominal pain invariably gets a CT scan. It may be precautionary, self-protective, and possibly help the patient. However, I do want to caution you that

CT scans carry very high levels of radiation that are dangerous to you and their cavalier usage may not be as benign as you are led to believe.

Testing Regimen for Patients Seeking Hormone Therapies

Balancing natural/human identical hormones in wellness and disease prevention focuses primarily on symptom relief. There are no firm guidelines for blood testing that correlate blood levels to real hormone balance. Saliva testing has not been proven to be of help either clinically or scientifically. Ultrasound is the only test that shows the effect of hormones on the uterine lining. For your treatments to be successful you must find a doctor who has solid experience in conventional and integrative medicine to help figure out what steps and tests are appropriate for you. Extremes don't work. Choose wisely and choose carefully.

Maria was 38 when she came to see me. She traveled from another city having read *The Hormone Solution* and, being proactive, she wanted to know how to stay ahead of problems that could be prevented, while taking full responsibility for the outcome in her life.

We worked together for a decade. She went through the usual transitions in her late 30s and 40s, she took progesterone for PMS, supplements to help stabilize her moods, and gradually changed her diet to a healthier vegetable-based one, low in animal fat, high in antioxidants (berries, dark, leafy green vegetables, and alkaline water and foods) to reduce inflammation. She exercised regularly and raised three wonderful children, even helped her physician husband understand the concept of true prevention and became a minister tending to the emotional needs of people in her congregation. Maria's progress was magnificent. She understood her body and as time passed, she became a highly aware empowered woman.

At the age of 49, Maria suddenly stopped having periods. It all coincided with her youngest son going to college and her parents selling the family childhood home and moving to South Carolina. I am sure many of you know exactly how this happens all at once. The life you led and thought you had under control suddenly changes and everything is new and different. You have to figure out who you are in this new body without hormones and full of new emotions. Maria was a trooper and I made sure our conversations delved into her personal life and the difficulties of dealing with so many sudden changes coinciding with the menopausal transition, all at the same time. While estradiol and progesterone helped balance her hormones we managed to help her adjust to her new life not only by balancing her hormones but also by providing a supportive, reassuring and kind ear.

Maria went to a local gynecologist in her town to have her routine annual PAP smear. The gynecologist conducted a thorough examination and found a few thyroid nodules. Maria had been on thyroid supplementation for a low thyroid I had diagnosed more than five years earlier. It isn't unusual for benign thyroid nodules to form when the thyroid slows down. The gynecologist decided to send her for a thyroid ultrasound. I thought the decision was sound. Unfortunately, that isn't where it all ended. The gynecologist also recommended Maria go to a local endocrinologist and stop taking the hormones I had been prescribing, even though Maria felt great and told that to the doctor. The doctor also told Maria to stop seeing me because my office wasn't in her town. He also told her seeing me twice a year and speaking to me on the phone or Facetime, even if it was weekly when she needed me, would not be enough. The doctor told Maria all hormone preparations were the same, and as a gynecologist she knew exactly what to do.

After she stopped taking the hormones and the thyroid for a while, Maria realized the doctor didn't really give her good care. She felt tired and no longer was thriving as she did under my care for more than a decade. She decided to come back to our practice and never returned to the doctor.

It may not be that the doctor was a bad doctor. Sadly, Maria's story is one I hear a lot. Doctors don't listen to the patients and let their egos get in the way of good care. I don't understand why doctors are competitive and ego-driven. I see them changing medications and giving contradictory advice for no good reason. In this case, the patient was doing well under my care for many years. All the doctor had to do was connect with me if she thought the patient would benefit from a change in her regimen. But the truth is, this wasn't about helping the patient. Sadly, it rarely is. It is time for doctors to remember they chose the medical profession to help people, not inflate their own egos. If your doctor does not listen to you I strongly suggest you follow Maria's example and just leave them. They will harm you in the long run and there are plenty of good doctors you can choose from. (Please read my book *Don't Let Your Doctor Kill You*, published by Post Hill Press, 2015.)

To help patients deal with conflicting information and provide them safe and reasonable follow-up I advise the following testing regimen (while keeping in mind that every person is different and care must be tailored to the individual patient's need by a caring and knowledgeable doctor):

- ▶ Baseline mammogram between ages 40 to 50 for women without family history of cancer or BRCA genetic mutations.
- ▶ Baseline comprehensive blood testing including hormone levels and breakdown of lipoproteins at the initial visit and then based on individual needs and symptoms on a bi-yearly or yearly basis.
- ▶ CIMT for all men and women over age 50.
- ▶ Pap smear yearly for menstruating women with multiple sex partners and every other year for women who have

stopped their menses. After the age of 55 this guideline must be reviewed based on individual patient situation, such as frequency of sexual activity, number of partners, and so forth. There may be no need to do Pap smears anymore at some point in our lives.

▶ Baseline screening bone density on women over 45. Repeat as desired by the patient if the family history suggests high risk for osteoporosis or the patient feels the need to know the state of her bones or is NOT taking estrogen regularly.

▶ Ultrasound of pelvis at the initial evaluation and yearly for all patients on hormone therapies.

▶ Baseline colonoscopy for women over 50 with no family history of colon cancer.

Before undertaking *any* test, ask yourself and the doctor: what will we do with the results of the test? If the results will affect course of treatment, by all means do it. If you are just doing the tests to say you did them, think twice.

...

CHAPTER 9

Understanding the Connection Between Hormones and Cancer

Hormones are very powerful molecules. Not all hormones have the same molecular structure thus they work differently in the body.

As a conventional physician, I was trained that estrogen—the hormone our body makes—and all estrogen substitutes were similar enough to be interchangeable. The reason for this belief comes from incorrect physician education. Medical school trains us that estrogen replacement for menopause consists exclusively of what is known as synthetic, but really means nonhuman identical, hormones. Although data questioning the safety and the efficacy of nonhuman identical hormone replacement abound in the medical literature, nothing about natural/bioidentical or human identical hormones is taught.

Let's spend a little time making sure we do understand the significance of this life-defining difference once and for all.

Estrogen

Estrogen is the name given to the hormones made by the ovaries, fat cells and adrenals of every human and mammal. It defines female characteristics and has a wide array of effects. As early as the late 1890s, women were given dried pregnant women's urine to help eliminate symptoms of menopause. By the 1930s estrogen was extracted from the urine of pregnant Canadian women. Menopausal women treated experienced remarkable results. Once treated with estrogen older women felt rejuvenated. As the demand for estrogen increased, the cost and availability of pregnant women's urine became prohibitive. So in the 1940s, stallions became the source for estrogen. That was because their urine contained high quantities of estrogen metabolites. Sadly, stallions could not be contained in stalls and harvesting their urine proved impossible. As a consequence, pregnant mares entered the world of hormone production. Wyeth, which owned a couple of pharmacies in both Canada and the U.S., started extracting estrogen from pregnant mares' urine, patented it, and named it Premarin (Pre-pregnant-Ma-mare-RIN-urine). (Look up "Premarin mares" on YouTube.)

The marketing and promotion of Premarin as the magic pill started in the 1950s but reached the tipping point in 1966 with the publication of Robert Wilson's book *Feminine Forever*. Dr. Wilson was paid $50,000 by Wyeth for the book, which became an immense success and launched Premarin as the drug bringing in the highest revenue in the history of big pharma. The drug helped immensely women desperate to stay young and attractive as well as free of menopausal symptoms. As a result of a highly successful marketing campaign the lay public and physicians alike (in academia or on Main Street, in little or huge practices, internists and ob/gyns) began to identify estrogen with Premarin.

Premarin and estrogen became just like Kleenex and tissues, Pampers and diapers. Thus the difference between the estrogen made by our bodies and the estrogen obtained from the pregnant horses' urine disappeared.

Since Premarin is a patented FDA-approved drug making hundreds of millions of dollars for its manufacturer (Wyeth pharmaceuticals at the time), the company's marketing engine squashed both the promotion and the study of other formulations of HRT. Over the course of the following three decades, estrogen replacement therapy became synonymous with Premarin in the U.S. As a consequence, the training of conventional doctors blurred and eventually eliminated any distinction between various forms of estrogen. The mainstream medical establishment barely addressed menopause and when doing so, left physicians with pseudo-scientific information while burying the real scientific data demonstrating the differences among hormones. Thus, natural/ bioidentical/human-identical/estradiol/17-betaestradiol-hormones weren't considered different from Premarin, even though they were well-studied. In fact, women treated with bioidenticals since the 1940s did consistently better than those on Premarin. Ignored was the fact that science supported their superior clinical results and gentle action in the human body for decades. The difference between their action and that of Premarin included safer bleeding parameters, cardiac sparing, improved lipid profile, lower cancer risk, and more. The pseudoscience bunched all hormones together and attributed the same effects to all.

Hopefully by the end of this chapter, I will have helped you understand the significant differences among the different preparations and types of hormones available on the market today so we can do away with the dogma that all hormones are the same.

Natural/bioidentical/human identical estrogen was not studied in the WHI meaning the data from that study does *not* apply to bioidentical hormones.

When I mention estrogen, I only refer to the hormone naturally made by our bodies- 17-beta estradiol, not the drugs obtained from pregnant mares' urine, or Premarin (also known as conjugated equine estrogen). Estrogen, human estrogen, defines us as women. It makes our breasts grow, it brings on our periods, it makes the lining of the uterus grow, it makes us ovulate, and it prepares and supports pregnancy and the growth of the fetus inside our wombs. It also protects us from heart disease, keeps our spirits high, raises serotonin levels, gives us energy, improves sleep quality, keeps our bones strong, and our metabolism in high gear.

Mother Nature ensures the perpetuation of the human species by revving up our bodies' hormone production. When we are young our bodies manufacture lots of estrogen in order to fulfill our physiologic mandate. High levels of estrogen bathe our every organ during pregnancy. These high levels of estrogen do not make us sick; as a matter of fact, they make us glow and keep us healthy. No pharmaceutical company would have endeavored to create an estrogen-like substance (trying to duplicate the effects of the natural molecule) if estrogen had been perceived as dangerous.

When Robert Wilson's book was published in 1966, estrogen was already established as the hormone that kept women healthy and able to multiply.

Birth Control Pills

Even though we've known that estrogen is a magnificent hormone since the beginning of the 20th century, scientists used our knowledge of estrogen to prevent women from getting pregnant. Birth control pills were developed in the 1930s, to stop women from ovulating, thus preventing pregnancies.

Birth control pills are ubiquitous (more than 10 million women are taking them), and every gynecologist pushes pills at every teen the second they walk through their office door, whether for acne, irregular periods, or menstrual cramps. The problem is that while we have gotten to a fourth generation of birth control pills, the dangers of using these drugs, which are hormone suppressors that stop the natural function of our entire endocrine system is totally overlooked and its dangers minimized in the medical literature and by clinicians.

Birth control pills were tried out in Nazi Germany during WWII in concentration camps to sterilize women as part of experimentation. Not a great start for the most commonly used tool in the battle against teen pregnancy in our public health system. Regardless of the fact that your gynecologist most likely will tell you birth control pills are safe, side-effects of birth control pills are numerous and should not be ignored. From mood swings, depression, and loss of libido to blood clots, cancer, infertility, and death, too many women suffer under our watch while the manufacturers of birth control pills refuse to allow the truth to come out.

Erica Langhart would be 28 today. Unfortunately, she died on Thanksgiving Day 2011 of a massive pulmonary embolus (a blood clot to her lungs) as a direct consequence of NuvaRing (third-generation birth control method along with Yaz, Yasmin, and Ortho Evra). Erica was a healthy 24-year-old when she suddenly developed shortness of breath and died within hours. Her physicians told her parents the death was caused by a blood clot to her lungs caused by the sudden release of high-dose synthetic nonhuman identical hormone into her bloodstream from NuvaRing. As a result, Erica's clotting mechanism was activated and her body made clots that traveled to her lungs and led to her untimely and tragic death.

Third-generation contraceptives like NuvaRing were the subject of a congressional hearing a month after Erica's death in December 2011. The panel of physicians who voted to keep these drugs on the market was made up of consultants to drug companies. Sadly, the media didn't cover the hearings. Unless you personally were negatively impacted by birth control pills, you don't have any way of knowing about the removal of Ortho Evra from the market or the many deaths caused by these medications.

I would not have known either if Erica's mother hadn't contacted me. She gave enough information to fill more than one book about the horrors associated with the birth control pill industry, how the truth about them is hidden from the public while young women' lives are endangered every day.

I will not go any further in this book with Erica's story or the story of birth control pills. I just want you to know that birth control pills are dangerous, they harm women, and they are made of the type of hormones that suppress our natural hormone production mechanisms, essentially leaving young women who use them functioning with the hormone levels of a woman in menopause. I recommend you read the book *Sweetening the Pill* by Holly Griggs-Spall to help provide a better perspective on the reality of this dangerous method of contraception. No bioidentical or natural hormone can be used for contraception because they don't suppress the body's natural function. Conversely, no nonhuman identical pills can be used when working with IVF and trying to get women pregnant.

The women who took Premarin in the 1960s (around 7 to 10 million) didn't offer significant complaints to their doctors to cause them to discontinue their use or seek alternative hormone preparations. When I started working with women in perimenopause in the mid-1980s, Premarin was the universal solution for all symptoms of menopause: hot flashes, night sweats, insomnia, mood swings, and even weight gain.

But then menopause was not a widely discussed topic until very recently. It was the WHI study that changed the landscape of HRT. Oddly, even today I still meet women in their mid- to late-50s who tell me they are not menopausal and have regular periods. Why are women still ashamed of menopause and afraid to tell the truth?

In the 1960s a woman's role was very much limited to the home, having and raising children, and very few ventured into the workforce. The women's movement was just beginning, and its leaders were more concerned with freedom to have sex without fear of pregnancy rather than long-term health, financial equality, and the long view of what happens at and after menopause. Most women didn't even know menopause existed. Our mothers never talked about it; I never even knew my mother went through menopause and I was a doctor. I remember hearing about a distant great-aunt who went crazy in mid-life and ended up in a mental institution, but no connection was ever made between mental or physical problems, loss of hormones, and menopause. Menopause was relegated to a deep, dark secret best not discussed. So without public outcry, with women compliantly following what the doctor tells them, the pharmaceutical companies just made, marketed, and sold drugs and Premarin stayed the only option for symptoms rarely discussed even in the doctor's office. And since it was heavily promoted to the doctors who had and still do have *no* medical training in menopause, Premarin became the market leader.

Premarin contains more than 200 estrogen-like molecules including equilenin and equilin, which are estrogens specific to the horse, completely foreign to our bodies. When molecules like equilenin and equilin attach to our cellular receptors, our immune system tries to fight it off. Our body defends itself from foreign molecules (horse protein in this case) by insulating the foreign molecule, by building walls around it or creating a systemic immune response. The wall may be a tumor or an abscess; the immune response could cause allergies, migraines or rashes. At a cellular level, the reaction is even more dramatic. Two scientific studies published in 1998 and 1999 in *Chemical Research in Toxicology* and *Proceedings of the Society for Experimental Biology and Medicine* proved without question that equilenin, once broken down in our bodies, becomes toxic to our own DNA.

By the early 1970s studies connected Premarin to increased incidence of uterine lining overgrowth and even uterine cancer. At the same times studies on birth control pills connected them to increased incidence of blood clots (to the legs and lungs). The situation caused concern and prompted a flurry of search for alternatives. Lower-dose estrogen birth control pills were developed although the basic make-up of birth control pills has remained the same to this day, synthetic/nonhuman identical hormones, which are the sole drugs that can suppress ovulation and prevent pregnancy.

As this was happening in the 1970s, I was in medical school and distinctly remember seeing patients with side-effects of these nonhuman identical estrogens (hormone impostors, hormone drugs) described in credible, sound, scientific articles. In the clinics of Kings County Hospital in Brooklyn, New York, where I trained, I saw women with swollen breasts, heavy irregular periods, ovarian cysts, phlebitis (inflamed, infected legs), thrombi (blood clots), and pulmonary embolisms (blood clots to the lungs). They were the living, breathing proof of the effects of synthetic estrogens reported in the medical literature. With all good intentions, we had started these patients on these nonhuman identical/synthetic hormones and suddenly were faced with unexpected consequences. We never made the connection between these problems and side-effects because we weren't taught about them in medical school or postgraduate training.

We were still in the honeymoon phase between pharmaceuticals and conventional, disease-centered medicine. The last thing the industry needed was for us to question its motives or its products.

In the time since the honeymoon ended and a long marriage ensued, many questions arose that cried out to be answered. As the data on significant side-effects of synthetic/nonhuman identical hormones appeared in the medical and lay literature, women and even doctors started to question their safety. Some stopped taking Premarin and birth control pills. Some were afraid to disobey their doctors. Many are still scared to tell their doctors of problems they are having with the medications, while too many just ignore the side-effects and live with their consequences no matter how dire or how easily avoidable.

Others with the guidance of physicians turned to the other hormones—bioidenticals/natural/human identicals for help with hormone balance.

Progesterone to Balance Estrogen

Pharmaceutical companies did not waste time cashing in on the need for progesterone once it became clear that Premarin alone had detrimental effects on the lining of the uterus. While progesterone is the natural hormone that balances estrogen's natural effect to make the lining of the uterus grow, progesterone is bioidentical and occurs in nature, thus unlikely to be patented. So just like with Premarin, a molecule similar to progesterone but not identical to it was created pharmaceutically to balance the effect of Premarin on the uterine lining and be patented and lucrative. Provera, Prempro, and Premphase were created. The fact is, bioidentical/human identical progesterone would have easily solved the problem of increased risk of endometrial cancer from Premarin, but a patented drug is much more financially rewarding. Provera isn't progesterone and creates terrible confusion for the public and medical profession. Provera (medroxyprogesterrone acetate) has side-effects similar to the pill (clotting problems) and may even cause cancer.

The point is that when you have the option of taking bioidentical hormones—hormones identical to those our bodies make—why would you take something that isn't identical? It's not even a matter of science, it's just common sense.

Hormones Not Identical to Human Hormones

- Premarin (pills) –Conjugated equine estrogen
- Menest (pills)
- Estratab (pills)
- Ogen (pills or cream)

- ▶ Ortho-Est (pills)
- ▶ Amen (pills)
- ▶ Aygestin (pills)
- ▶ Curretab (pills)
- ▶ Cycrin (pills)
- ▶ Depo Provera–Medroxyprogesterone acetate (injectable)
- ▶ Norlutate (pills)
- ▶ Provera (pills)

Combinations

- ▶ Prempro (pills)
- ▶ Premphase (pills)
- ▶ CombiPatch (patch)

All Birth Control Pills and Other Forms of Birth Control Contain Non-Human Identical Hormones

All the above are drugs manufactured to fool our bodies into believing we are getting the hormones we desperately need. Some of them have been removed from the market while others still sell. Unfortunately, these hormones cannot fool our cells because they don't fit into their cellular receptors and cause undesirable side-effects:

1. Replace and inactivate whatever hormones our bodies produce by blocking receptors and sending messages to the pituitary gland to stop our own hormone production.
2. Change the normal configuration of receptors, confusing the cells and stimulating defensive immune responses. In the short run, they may create loss of libido, weight gain, sleep disturbances, mood changes, irritability,

palpitations, anxiety, depression, and other symptoms.
In the long run, they may cause infertility, depression,
weight gain, insulin resistance, suppression of thyroid and
adrenals, cancers, blood clots, and heart disease.

When synthetic/nonhuman identical hormone replacement became popular in the mid-1960s, the long-term effects could not be anticipated, but many telltale signs of their incompatibility with the human body were noticed early on. Unfortunately, most women taking them either ignored the side-effects, didn't make the connection between the medications and the side-effects or went off the medications and never shared important information with their doctors. Whether informed or not, the FDA didn't address the problems. The drug companies are required to report adverse reactions to the FDA. The incentive is minimal because reporting problems would lead to diminished income. What would you think the likelihood of these reports making it to the FDA are?

I remember feeling sick the first month I took birth control pills at the age of 19. I was placed on them because I had severe menstrual cramps. My doctor told me "they would eliminate my cramps and as an added bonus they would protect me from getting pregnant." He didn't even ask if I was sexually active. Within three weeks I had migraines, became bloated and moody and felt like I was living in another person's body. I called my doctor and asked if my new symptoms could be connected to the birth control pills. He told me it was very unlikely. I stopped taking birth control pills after two months when one morning I failed to recognize my best friend in front of my apartment and the symptoms persisted. I never went back to that doctor, nor did I call to tell him what happened.

When I went into private practice, I listened to similar complaints from many healthy young women on birth control pills. When they complained of headaches I gave them painkillers, when bloated I gave them diuretics. When they lost their libido I had no idea what to do. It took years for me to make the connection between birth control pills and its multitude of side-effects. And then it took another few years to realize the best treatment is to discontinue the use of the birth control pills rather than to treat their side-effects. I find that in general if a woman reacts to one type of birth control pill, her chances of tolerating others are minimal. I don't like to suggest any synthetic/nonhuman identical hormones to help with birth control (I recommend Paragard IUD without hormones). Long-term side-effects of birth control pills may include infertility, cancer and premature ovarian failure which leads to early menopause. Most are not being addressed because birth control pills are useful in preventing teen pregnancy, which is a major public health issue. The medical literature offers no research, no data and no transparency about birth control pills. It is odd that no studies are being published on the long-term effects of birth control pills, when they are the number one hormonal method of contraception in use for the past 50 years.

Endometrial/Uterine Cancer and Premarin

Estrogen causes the lining of the uterus to grow in healthy women. Progesterone counteracts unchecked growth stimulated by estrogen. Progesterone makes cells stop growing. Thus, it prevents overgrowth of the lining of the uterus, aka endometrium. Uterine cancer is a rare disease in the general population. According to the National Cancer Institute it represents 1.8 percent of all cancer deaths in 2016. This disease was brought to us largely through HRT treatments with synthetic/nonhuman identical estrogens.

Between the 1950s when Premarin came to the market and the 1970s when the data on endometrial cancer started to appear in the medical literature, hundreds of thousands of women were treated with Premarin alone without progesterone.

In the mid-1970s, studies making the connection between Premarin and increased incidence of endometrial cancer started to appear in the medical journals. The results of the studies showed that women who took nonhuman identical estrogen for 1-5 years had a three-fold increase in incidence of uterine cancer. Those who took the nonhuman identical estrogen for 10 years had a 10-fold increase. Lifetime use of synthetic/nonhuman identical estrogen alone potentially increased a woman's chance of getting uterine cancer to 1 in 10.

During my medical training in the mid to late 1970s, we were taught that although the incidence of deaths from uterine cancer had increased twofold to threefold in the years since Premarin became the main estrogen replacement therapy, uterine cancer was a low-grade cancer. (Brinton LA, Hoover RN. and the Endometrial Cancer Collaborative Group. Estrogen replacement therapy and endometrial cancer risk: unresolved issues. *Obstet Gynecol.* 1993;81:265–271.) By 1993 studies found that uterine cancer caused by treatment with Premarin had a 90 percent cure rate as compared to uterine cancer in general, with a cure rate of only 70 to 75 percent. This may sound good to a statistician but it sounded plain wrong to me. I went into medicine to protect my patients, not choose the least of two evils for them, or hide behind statistics. My professors of obstetrics and gynecology were quick to point out that as soon as we figured out the need to balance estrogen (synthetic/nonhuman identical estrogen) with progestin (synthetic/nonhuman identical progestin), the risk of developing uterine cancer was practically eliminated. Unfortunately, they were right in theory; but in practice we were not balancing with progesterone, we were balancing with yet another foreign nonhuman identical hormone.

As a young doctor desperately wanting to help my patients and believing in the system that educated me, I took the information to heart and started every symptomatic menopausal patient on the new combination Prempro, Premphase or cycled Premarin, and Provera.

But, as a precaution my patients also had annual pelvic ultrasounds. Premarin took away the hot flashes and Provera reassured me it would protect my patients from endometrial cancer even though they seemed to develop never-ending periods. I thought that was good. I was in my 20s and did not know that 55-year-old women don't need to have a period.

By the mid-1990s many studies addressed the combination of medroxyprogesterone acetate (Provera) and conjugated equine estrogen (Premarin) and the good and bad effects on women's uteruses, breasts, bleeding profiles and cholesterol levels. While factually the information gathered from these studies is true—unopposed estrogen therapy may increase the risk of uterine cancer—no alternative, safe and human identical solution was offered except in one study, the PEPI trials, that showed that women taking Premarin with progesterone, the natural hormone, fared better in all parameters studied than women taking nonhuman identical progestins (medroxyprogesterone acetate, or Provera).

Since natural/bioidentical/human identical hormones were not included in the large studies of the 1990s the situation left a very important question unanswered: was the increased rate of endometrial cancer caused by all estrogen or by nonhuman identical estrogen specifically?

Let's not forget another piece of information research uncovered: estrogen, the hormone made by our body, has practically no connection with endometrial cancer. The average woman who has never taken hormone replacement (HRT) practically never gets endometrial cancer. It occurs in less than 1 in 1,000 women each year according to a 1998 report in the American Journal of Obstetrics and Gynecology. This number is based only on information obtained from women who have pelvic examinations. Fewer than 10% of women in the population at-large do.

Ovarian Cancer

On March 21, 2001, the *Journal of the American Medical Association* reported on a 15-year study conducted by the American Cancer Society. The study determined that women who took estrogen replacement (Premarin, Prempro, Provera) for more than 10 years between 1982 to 1996 had double the normal risk of dying from ovarian cancer.

Within 48 hours of its publication, the data reviewed by academic medical centers and the media was deemed statistically insignificant, and the study flawed. Unfortunately, the information, albeit discarded, raised another question about the dangers of synthetic/non-human identical estrogen replacement therapy.

LouAnn died of ovarian cancer at 46 in 1996. She was single, had no children, and had been taking Prempro for 15 years because her doctor told her it would help prevent osteoporosis, which was prevalent in her family. When she became my patient, she had already been diagnosed with ovarian cancer and had undergone surgery and chemotherapy. Nothing worked. I provided more hospice care for her than medical care. Sadly, I watched her wither away and die without much more than kindness to offer.

After the publication of the ovarian cancer study in 2001, I could not help but wonder about LouAnn. Yes, she was at higher risk of getting ovarian cancer because she didn't have children. But, who could tell if the 15 years she took Prempro didn't contribute or push her over the edge? For me, LouAnn was not just another statistic, she was a young woman whose death was another strike against synthetic/non-bioidentical estrogen replacement therapy.

Breast Cancer

Although 80 percent of women who get breast cancer don't have common risk factors, contributory factors like genetics, stress, lifestyle, environmental and those caused by our overly aggressive and harsh treatments must be given serious consideration. We are exposed to chemicals and phytoestrogens in the environment and foods containing nonhuman identical estrogens, we eat meat and vegetables treated with synthetic hormones and radiation and then we take them willingly in the form of birth control or menopausal treatments that are synthetic/nonhuman identical estrogen replacement therapy. In 1990, an article entitled "The Endocrinology of Breast Cancer" published in *Cancer* established a significant connection between continuous exposure to nonhuman identical estrogen and the development of breast cancer. Since then, studies on synthetic/nonhuman identical estrogens and the constant avalanche of fear mongering media and medical marketing have only served to increase the panic women experience living with the possibility of developing breast cancer. Even though breast cancer is not the number one killer of women, its connection to hormone replacement therapy remains the main deterrent for use of HRT. Unfortunately, the fact that natural/human identical progesterone and estrogens offer protection from breast cancer as proven by study after study (see references) has been overshadowed by the negative publicity received by their synthetic counterparts and the marketing of breast cancer as a disease women must fear more than heart disease, which is the real killer of aging women deprived of hormone therapies.

▶ The KEEPS/Kronos study conducted between 2002 and 2012 found favorable effects with hormones in menopausal women. Oral Premarin and human identical Climara patch were compared for the first time in a study that looked at young women for a short period of time. The results failed to show a difference between synthetic and bio-identicals because the dose was very low in both products and the time period studied too short. However, the study did prove CIMT an optimum test to use to establish the presence of heart disease. And no participant got cancer in the period of time studied, debunking some of the connection between HRT and cancer.

▶ The results of a Danish study, a randomized study released in 2013, that looked at more than 10,000 women who took bioidentical/human-identical hormones for 10 years found that women on high doses of oral bioidentical hormones (estradiol 4 mg/day) had a lower risk of heart disease, stroke, cancer, and thromboembolism than those not taking hormones.

▶ Race differences and country of residence are significant. Caucasian Americans over the age of 45 are most likely to be diagnosed with breast cancer. This is a function of statistics. In African American women breast cancer has poorer prognosis and earlier age peak of incidence. The types of breast cancer African American women develop are more virulent and occur in younger women. Research specifically on breast cancer in African American women is largely inexistent. Aging American women of middle to higher socio-economic levels have more mammograms, more regular check-ups and are targeted by the media for all types of breast cancer awareness activities. Asian women have a very low incidence of breast cancer and scientists are in constant debate over the reasons why. Genetics are an obvious factor but there is much more we do not know. And statistics won't help us.

▶ Regarding family history of breast cancer, BRCA (Breast Cancer) 1 and 2 genes account for 80 percent of inherited cancer cases. Other genes including HER2 and p53 account for other genetically inherited breast cancers. It is important to realize that more than 40 percent of women with these genetic mutations do not get cancer by the age of 70. BRCA genes, in the instances they are expressed, are associated with breast, ovarian and colon cancer in women, and prostate and colon cancer in men. Jews of Eastern European origin carry these genes at a 2.3 percent rate. The population at-large has less than 0.003 percent chance of carrying these genes. FORCE (Facing Our Risk of Cancer Empowered, at www.facingourrisk.org) and provide important communication and support for women carrying these genes. Keep in mind that all statistics provided are based on the women who are diagnosed and go for the tests. This means the statistics NEVER represent the reality of the population at-large. We have no idea what the real numbers are because most women do not have the tests.

▶ Looking at the personal history of breast cancer, women who have had breast cancer have a fivefold chance of getting breast cancer again in the opposite breast or the same breast. You already know a history of multiple breast biopsies increases the risk of breast cancer. Scar tissue is formed at the site of the biopsy and the risk of developing cancer in scar tissue has been under investigation by researchers for years. Not to be forgotten is the fact that biopsies alter the immune system's reaction while also changing the anatomy of the breast and thus opening the door for unexpected and unresearched spread.

▶ Blind biopsies used to be the norm for evaluation of fibrocystic breasts. Although no sound connection between fibrocystic breasts and cancer exists, to this day it is not unusual to hear about doctors doing needle biopsies in their office to quickly diagnose the make-up of a possible mass. In my opinion, no woman should ever allow a doctor to blindly perform an aspiration biopsy. The only acceptable method of evaluating breast masses is the stereotactic biopsy procedure (see Chapter 8). And even that must be for suspected real cancers, not slowly growing ones like DCIs (ductal carcinoma in situ), which is even a questionable cancer due to its slow progression and cytological features.

▶ Then there are environmental factors. Chemicals, antibiotics and hormones are part of our lives: exposure to PCBs (polychlorinated bisphenyls) in our rivers, DDT (insecticide) sprays, DES (diethylstilbestrol), and other hormones fed to our farm animals (in doses so high no human would ever be prescribed), high voltage electricity in our backyard, and chemical and radiation pollution are undoubtedly contributing factors to clusters of breast cancer outbreaks. I strongly recommend you watch two documentaries that will change the way you see and possibly eat food for the rest of your life: *Food, Inc.* and *Forks Over Knives.*

▶ Women on high animal-fat diets are also at risk. Women of European, South American and North American descent where high intake of animal fat is a common staple are at higher risk of breast cancer. These women produce more estrogen (estrogen made in fat cells) than women whose diet is mostly vegetable and grain. The statistical difference for the incidence of breast cancer is significant. For more information on how diet affects risk of chronic illnesses including breast cancer please read *The China Study*. I strongly encourage women to change their diets to high fiber, organic vegetables, minimum animal fat, no dairy, no processed sugar, no alcohol, and *no* smoking.

Before I conclude on the topic of breast cancer I want to bring in another related topic—the use of designer estrogens or anti-estrogen drugs.

The Estrogen Window Hypothesis on Breast Cancer

An interesting and common-sense theory on the development of breast cancer is called the Estrogen Window Hypothesis, circulated for more than two decades in the alternative medicine world although its origin comes from conventional medicine. According to this theory, breast cancer often starts during the 10-15 years before menopause. It is during this period of time that estrogen is dominant in our bloodstream. As you recall from Chapter 1, the quality and quantity of progesterone we make decreases with age. Hence we live in an estrogen-dominated environment for many years before menopause. According to the Estrogen Window Hypothesis, it is during this time that, unbalanced by progesterone, breast tissue cells keep growing under the stimulation of our own internal estrogen production. Considering the average rate of doubling time for breast cancer cells at 3-6 months, we have 8-10 years to get to the diagnosable-level (be it mammogram or palpation) size tumor.

If women start supplementing with natural, micronized progesterone during those 8–10 years before menopause, we could possibly help save many women from breast cancer. What is the downside of micronized progesterone supplementation? None to date. And that's with more than 30 years of wide usage as of 2016. For more, read "Oestrogen Window Hypothesis of the Aetiology of Breast Cancer" in *Lancet* 1:700-701, 1980.

Designer Estrogens—SERMs

SERMs—Selective estrogen receptor modulators—are a group of drugs that compete with human estrogen for specific sites on cell receptors. They are synthetic/nonhuman identical; in fact, they have nothing to do with hormones and are designed to replace estrogen in certain tissues. They bind to estrogen-alpha and beta receptors and together they form a complex structure with varying effects on human organs.

On uterus and bones, the complex has estrogen-like effects, but on breast tissue it has an anti-estrogen effect. SERMs are designed to protect women from increased risk of estrogen-positive breast cancer and endometrial cancer. In fact, SERMs are given to women who have had breast cancers for up to seven years after the cancer has been removed and much research work seems to point toward some minimal benefit, but the side-effects far outweigh the benefits.

The two most commonly used are raloxifene (Evista) and tamoxifen (Nolvadex). A special report published in March 2001 in the *Journal of Postgraduate Medicine* through a grant of Merck & Co. Inc., provides an overview on The Effects of SERMs on Women's Health (www.ncbi.nlm.nih.gov/pubmed/11296735). The report raises questions of safety of use, risk-benefit ratio and overall increases of dangerous side-effects. Today, more than 15 years after that report, most oncologists still prescribe these drugs in spite of serious doubts about their effectiveness and safety. New small studies and reviews of studies crop up periodically encouraging the use of these drugs for cancer prevention yet no one addresses the horrific effects they have on women's quality of life.

Tamoxifen

The National Surgical Adjuvant Breast and Bowel P-1 trial regarding tamoxifen therapy for breast cancer concluded that:

- ▶ Tamoxifen significantly decreased the relative risk of breast cancer by 49 percent.
- ▶ Follow-up on tamoxifen's impact on overall mortality was not available. The authors of the study strongly recommended it be made available.
- ▶ **Trial results do not apply to the population at-large**.
- ▶ Tamoxifen was not recommended for the prevention of osteoporosis. Women over the age of 50, who are at highest risk of breast cancer, had the most adverse effects.

> ▶ The benefits did not outweigh the adverse effects (hot flashes, night sweats, insomnia, weight gain, palpitations, foggy thinking, depression, and more), which significantly affected the quality of life of women.

Tamoxifen is prescribed for a minimum of five years in women who have had breast cancer. It is prescribed prophylactically in women who don't have breast cancer but may be considered at risk. This treatment is based on the results of a National Cancer Institute study (WHEN) questioned repeatedly by English and Italian scientists in articles published in medical journals all over the world.

Tamoxifen is associated with a 2.5 to 7.5 times increased risk of uterine cancer. The types of uterine cancers associated with tamoxifen are more aggressive than any other. Tamoxifen is associated with increased incidence of blood clots, thrombophlebitis and pulmonary emboli. Tamoxifen induces early menopause and all its symptoms: weight gain, severe night sweats, hot flashes, depression, anxiety and loss of libido. Long-term effects include thinning bones (osteopenia and osteoporosis) and heart disease.

Once considered taboo, placing women on hormones after breast cancer appears to be safe now and the huge debate and arguments of 10 years ago among oncologists, gynecologists, and complementary doctors is subsiding among those who actually care about the patient and her quality of life. Leading from a position of care and kindness rather than fear and intimidation seems to bring confidence and women making decisions based on higher quality of life rather than fear of cancer.

Raloxifene

Raloxifene is another designer anti-estrogen drug with far-reaching medical implications. Its chemical make-up is very much similar to tamoxifen.

Raloxifene was initially developed to treat breast cancer as well. When during its trials it failed to produce a good therapeutic response, it was re-routed as an estrogen-like drug for the treatment of osteoporosis.

A study by Delmas and Ettinger concluded that raloxifene was effective in both prevention and treatment of postmenopausal osteoporosis and the FDA approved its use for those indications. Another role for raloxifene was found in its decrease of LDL cholesterol levels. Two studies *Raloxifene Use for the Heart* (RUTH, 2007) and *Multiple Outcomes of Raloxifene Evaluation* (MORE, 2001) found the following results:

- ▶ Raloxifene significantly decreased the relative risk of breast cancer by 76 percent in the population studied. Population studied does not mean everybody and relative risk doesn't mean absolute risk, which is the only risk that truly applies to the individual.
- ▶ Raloxifene increased the risk of deep vein thrombosis, pulmonary embolism and retinal vein thrombosis 3:1.
- ▶ Performance on cognitive function tests was not improved.
- ▶ LDL cholesterol was decreased, but HDL (good cholesterol) was not increased.
- ▶ Bone mineral density was only marginally increased.

Side-effects of raloxifene include hot flashes, night sweats, and bloating. It's of no help in treating hot flashes, improving good cholesterol, preventing heart disease, or preventing Alzheimer's.

Summary on Hormone Therapy Studies

Over the course of the past two decades that I have been working with hormones, I've had the pleasure of reviewing most of the conventional and integrative scientific literature on hormones in both men and women in health and disease. Studies that connect the use of estrogen to cancer in general invariably refer to the usage of synthetic/nonhuman identical estrogens. Even in that situation, the only statistically significant connection between use of synthetic/nonhuman identical estrogens and cancer has been made in the case of extended use of unopposed synthetic/nonhuman identical estrogens and uterine cancer.

Reassuring information comes to us from studies that reveal the combination of synthetic/nonhuman identical estrogens with synthetic/nonhuman identical progestins provide protection from uterine cancer. The problem with the nonhuman identical progestins above all is the alteration in bleeding parameters increasing the risk of blood clots and strokes as well as heart attacks.

After the demise of the WHI, Provera (medroxyprogesterone acetate) was deemed the bad guy and fell into disfavor. However, most gynecologists routinely use it even today to bring on late periods. Sadly, the situation only serves to demonstrate the level of up-to-date information most gynecologists have. We have so much scientific literature culminating with the most recent results of the KEEPS and Danish studies that demonstrate that natural/bioidentical hormones provide protection from heart disease, don't increase the risk of blood clots or Alzheimer's and do not increase the risk of either breast cancer or other chronic illnesses.

As the public understanding and search for natural/bioidentical hormones has increased dramatically over the past decade, education to raise physician awareness as well as training to provide unified safe and scientifically sound protocols for the use of natural/bioidentical/human identical hormones is cropping up outside the academic centers still mired in special interest games. (For more information please go to www.bhionline.org.)

CHAPTER 10

Diet, Exercise, Lifestyle, Telomeres, and Supplements

We waste an enormous amount of time trying to fit into the mold of beauty and youth created by the media. In the process, we lose ourselves or never get to know who we really are. Just look at the constant frenzy of features in magazines, ads, internet, and social media, all in constant search of the magic pill, magic diet, magic supplement to help us stay thin and forever young. There is no such thing as one magic solution. Human beings are so complex and unique, snake oil answers are just snake oil. Only good genetics and a well-balanced body and mind will keep us in decent health for our entire life.

Finally, it has become fact that ideal hormone balance is directly connected to optimum health regardless of age. With the aid of natural/bioidentical/human identical hormones, we can achieve excellent hormone balance and live symptom-free regardless of age. But proper hormone balance is not enough. As we go through life, we cannot overlook the significant contributions of diet, exercise, lifestyle, stress management, supplements, and even the role of our telomeres.

A couple of years ago, I had no trouble identifying my patients' ages. Today, as I work exclusively in the area of wellness and prevention I am no longer surprised by the youthful appearance of 65-year-olds who look 40 and who have no trace of chronic illnesses whatsoever.

While these people are taking natural/bioidentical/human identical hormones, they also follow an organic, low-processed sugar, minimal animal fat diet, exercise regularly, take telomerase inhibitors and supplements, meditate, sleep 7 to 8 hours every night, and follow excellent stress management programs.

The correct hormone balance opens the door to wellness and disease prevention. To stay healthy, you must capitalize on the opportunity hormones give you to change your diet, improve your exercise regimen, and get those much needed 7 to 8 hours of sleep a night, not to mention getting rid of all toxic relationships from your life. Then, you can truly say you have found the Fountain of Youth.

All success stories of people who feel and look great regardless of age over long periods of time have one thing in common—truly balanced lives. A little change in as many aspects of our lives as possible, brings about a logarithmic improvement in the quality of our lives as a whole.

I don't believe people should follow extreme programs, be it in exercise or diet. They don't work. What works is a little change at a time, giving yourself permission to follow your own rules and learning to accept yourself exactly as you are.

Diet

Nothing is more obvious than the fact that we are what we eat. And still we ignore this fact by eating junk. Americans are fatter than ever because we eat fast food, chow down while in the car, grab a bite between meetings, drink soda, caffeinated drinks, and alcohol in ever increasing quantities, and pretty much intentionally ignore the scientifically proven deadly details of our diets.

"JUNK IN, JUNK OUT." Based on this simple concept I believe that if you put junk food into your body, your body will spend its resources trying to process the junk and extract whatever little nutritional value from it, creating more junk (toxins, free radicals), weighing you down, and making you sick. **Eating junk speeds up aging.**

We need food to make fuel to keep our body systems working optimally. Fuel is energy. However, before food can be turned into fuel it must be broken down into very small useful particles that eventually become the raw materials to make energy. The factories to make energy are situated in every cell in our bodies and are called mitochondria. The process of breaking down food, absorbing the nutrients and making energy in the mitochondria is called metabolism and it is under the direct control of our hormones. I am sure you know and probably hate people with fast metabolisms who burn up every piece of cake they eat with impunity and never gain an ounce. I am also sure you know and feel sorry for people with slow metabolisms, those unfortunate souls who get fat just by looking at a piece of bread.

While genetics are important in determining who has a slow and who has a fast metabolism, hormones implement our genetic mandate. People with low thyroid, adrenal fatigue, and metabolic syndrome are typical examples of slow metabolizers. Less known is the fact that when estrogen and progesterone start waning, the metabolic rate goes down as well, and we start gaining weight. The connection between low thyroid and low estrogen and progesterone is finally coming to light in the conventional literature. Low thyroid is a common yet overlooked side-effect of birth control pills and any other hormone replacement that suppresses natural hormone production. When we supplement with bioidentical/human identical, adrenal and thyroid hormones we create a bulwark against aging that leads to metabolic slowdown. With the help of hormones, we start feeling better and should use that opportunity to clean up our diet, increase our physical activity, get more sleep, meditate, learn and apply stress management techniques and eliminate all negative thinking from our lives. That package will keep us healthy and thriving indefinitely.

Balancing Your Foods

The first step in the process of fine-tuning your eating habits is becoming aware of the food we eat. The food pyramid you learned in school is obsolete. Think of the "Food Balance" and "The Hormone Friendly Diet" instead. To achieve ideal balance in nutrition, the balance must tip the scale toward protein, vegetable fat and fiber and vegetables and berries and stay light on the sugar and animal fat side.

Natural/Organic Foods

When we refer to natural foods, we mean unprocessed, untreated, and also organic foods. But this whole concept is at odds with the conveniences created by modern age. How can we have plastic bags with sliced bread, cereal in boxes, frozen prepared foods in our grocery stores edible for months, and canned foods that last for years? The magic of chemical preservatives has affected us deeply and badly. Laden with chemicals, our processed foods may look good and taste wonderful to our polluted taste buds but lead to toxicity and a rapidly aging body. Our cells have no ability to detoxify and break down processed, chemical-filled, refined, artificial foods that make up so much of our standard diet. Our cells can only process nutrients from natural, organic foods. Just as with natural hormones, our body can only benefit from natural foods. Everything else creates more problems than it solves.

I tell my patients to just try eating unprocessed foods for a week or two. Invariably they tell me about the remarkable changes they experience in their energy level, the quality of their sleep, and their moods. So, why aren't we all turning to natural foods? The answer I often hear is, "I'm so busy with my life, it's more difficult to get healthy food than grab a candy bar, a bag of potato chips or a can of soda." Maybe that was true 10 years ago, but today that's no longer a good excuse. More people are aware of the importance of eating clean, natural, organic foods so learning to read labels is crucial. The rule of thumb is simple: if you cannot pronounce the ingredient on the label don't buy the product. I'm not suggesting you only eat organic, locally grown foods. I understand that may still be difficult and costly. Today most large chain supermarkets carry fresh foods, multigrain cereals, breads, nuts, fruit and organic meats. All you have to do is shop on the outside aisles and avoid the inner aisles where canned foods, soda and all chemical-filled stuff is. Why not start there? You'll feel the difference! I guarantee.

Get Off the Sugar Roller Coaster

Sugar seems to give us the energy boost we need in the middle of the afternoon or right before our period when progesterone and estrogen levels drop and fatigue becomes unbearable. The price we pay for eating sugars is much too high. Sugar—candy, candy bars, soda, chocolate, cake, any type of sweets, and prepared foods with added sugar—turn into glucose as it enters the bloodstream. Blood sugar levels rapidly rise. A sudden rush of energy follows and the exhausted, shaky, sweaty, hungry feeling disappears. The brain, now overflowing with sugar, sends a message to the pancreas to release insulin. Insulin is a hormone that causes blood sugar levels to drop, pushing the sugar into storage in the liver and fat cells. Blood sugar level drops like a lead balloon. Within a couple of hours of this vicious cycle, you feel drained and exhausted, shaky, sweaty, hypoglycemic. This is a never-ending roller coaster, because, whether you realize it or not, the same foods that made you hypoglycemic to begin with are the quick fix foods you crave. Sadly, these foods create an erosive and dangerous cycle of high sugar, rapid insulin release followed by low blood sugar, leaving you perpetually drained, fatigued, and sick.

Refined sugars may taste delicious in cakes, cookies, ice cream, bread, pizza, or pasta, but they are our worst enemies in the fight against weight gain, aging, and chronic illnesses. The only types of sugars that do not send you into the insulin/hypoglycemia cycle are protein and fat, fruit and vegetables. Nothing more, nothing less.

Fat Fads

Twenty years ago, low-fat diets were the fad. After the connection among high cholesterol, heart disease, and diets high in saturated fats was made, cardiologists and nutritionists placed all patients at risk of heart disease on low-fat diets. I was never keen on the idea because I noticed that people on low-fat diets were always hungry, fatigued, pasty looking, with thin hair and dry skin. Their cholesterol levels may have been low, but they sure looked sick. The problem with the low-fat diet is that it indiscriminately eliminated all fats from our diet, and cholesterol (a most important fat) is the precursor for all hormones. Low cholesterol is dangerous to our health.

Fat is very important in the maintenance of our cell membranes and contributes to our having shiny hair, strong nails, and smooth skin. Fat is a most important ingredient for healthy bodies and minds. It is essential for healthy brain and muscle function. Cholesterol is critical to the manufacture of all hormones. People on low-fat diets cannot make hormones and thus feel fatigued. I am not suggesting we all start eating bacon, heavy cream and fatty meats like diets prevalent in the 1990s did (e.g., Atkins). Just like sugars, the source and kind of fat determines if it is healthy or not. Animal fat from meat and dairy are saturated fats leading to increased risk of obesity and heart disease. (Remember The China Study and the documentary *Forks over Knives*.)

Another source of dangerous fats is margarine and hydrogenated oils, called trans-fatty acids, also directly connected to increased incidence of heart disease and breast cancer. The good fats are known as unsaturated fats and they are abundant in vegetables like avocado, olives, coconut, almonds, and so forth. Women who carry a few extra pounds do have an easier time with menopause because estrogen is stored in fat cells. You know that after a meal full of saturated fats you feel sluggish and want to take a nap. Not so if your meal contains mono- and polyunsaturated fats. Not only do they keep your energy up, they relieve PMS, decrease bad cholesterol, lower blood pressure, decrease the risk of heart attacks, and may even decrease the growth of breast cancer. Monounsaturated fats are found in olive oil, avocado, nuts, flaxseed, hemp, and fatty fish (salmon, mackerel, sardines). You can find good fats in supplement form most commonly as linoleic acid (omega-6) and linolenic acid (omega-3).

Weight Control

Any discussion about nutrition and diet invariably turns to weight loss. Obesity in the U.S. is at an all-time high. Most diets are based on the premise that if you put less food in your mouth (eat fewer calories) you will force your body to break down its fat stores and lose weight. Not quite true. Low-calorie diets without correct hormone support rob you of energy and leave you fatigued and depleted without helping you shed the pounds. I've developed "The Hormone Friendly Diet" (www.eshealth.com) over two decades of work with hormones with patients who are also looking for a way to lose weight. The results provide not only balanced

HCG Diet

In our practice, we often jump-start some of our patients with a short course of injectable HCG. First, we balance their hormones and then we help them lose 10 to 20 pounds rapidly by cutting down their caloric intake to 500 to 750 calories with the supplemental help of HCG (the hormone of pregnancy in very low doses). Carefully watching our patients, we achieve consistently great success with this combination and patients are happy with the results. The HCG hormone is very useful because during the acute weight loss phase it protects from developing unsightly loose skin by eliminating fat only and not losing the supportive connective tissue, making it look flexible and strong.

Please be careful with any diet and do not do it alone. Even if you change your eating habits for a while, if your hormones are not in proper balance, weight gain will continue and the time and effort you spent on dieting will be wasted. Disappointment is not in my vocabulary so I make sure everything we do in our offices makes patients happy and keeps them safe. That is why our nutritional support includes HCG diet and The Hormone Friendly Diet.

hormones but also the correct dietary support regardless of age. By increasing self-awareness eating a well-balanced diet becomes a way of life rather than a diet you follow for a while.

Portions: Size Matters

To give your cells the fuel to make good energy, to maintain hormone balance, to keep your blood sugar levels even, to keep insulin steady, small food portions at frequent intervals are most helpful tools. But please don't go crazy measuring and weighing your foods.

One of my patients, Laurie, a food critic, taught me to think of the way food is presented. She said to start by imagining a beautiful plate in a great restaurant. Then decide how much food you should pile on it. If you want to lose weight, fill half the plate. If you want to maintain, fill three-fourths. Never fill a full plate, and make sure its presentation is appealing. Never eat food that is not appealing because it won't satisfy you. Europeans and Asians are experts at portion control. You will never see them eating oversized or aesthetically unpleasing meals. Let's learn from them.

Group 1: Preliminary Symptoms

Age Group: Teens and Early 20s

It would be unrealistic and even cruel to expect a teen to eliminate McDonalds French fries, burgers, tacos, pizza, and soda from their diet. But unfortunately, some of the symptoms of hormone imbalance experienced by this age group are directly related to the high content of refined sugar, saturated fat, and trans-fat found in the fast foods that are staples for teens and young 20s.

Remember Michelle with the acne problem? Not only did she require topical antibiotics and natural progesterone supplementation to get rid of the acne, she also benefited from a dietary makeover. She loved soda. Often she had soda for breakfast, lunch, and dinner, and even in between. When she felt a little tired, she'd take a swig of the soda she carried with her wherever she went. Over a period of two months we weaned her off soda and taught her to drink water instead. While she still has an occasional soda fix, she only drinks it on special occasions. This change in her diet alone was crucial. Soda is full of caffeine, chemicals, and sugar. These substances only served to throw off her hormone balance and very likely added to her problem with acne.

You recall Louise with the mood swings? Turns out she was addicted to sugar, especially the week before her period. Her most severe mood swings coincided with nightly treats of frozen yogurt or ice cream. As a result, she had trouble sleeping and spent her days in brain fog and severe fatigue. Natural progesterone cream she applied to her inner arms at night before going to bed helped tame her sugar cravings. Connecting the severe changes in personality to her nocturnal food intake helped her stop the habit and eliminate the sugar fix. Louise still goes out for ice cream occasionally. Only now she does it during the day and mostly on weekends. Making the connection between cravings and hormone issues is very important. If your hormones are out of balance you will definitely crave sugar and fatty foods and they will make you sicker and more uncomfortable, creating a vicious circle you need to break.

Reasonable expectations must be the rule specifically for this age group. They are young, must be able to try different foods and enjoy life. But the earlier young people make the connection between symptoms and food intake, the quicker they improve their dietary intake and then feel better. Even if many teens get help from their parents, it is important for them to learn to balance their diets on their own. You don't want them to have to play catch-up in their 30s or later. Body awareness is a huge side-benefit of teaching proper eating habits early in life.

Encourage your children to eat a balanced diet high in proteins, vegetables, and fruit. As frequently as possible, have family dinners. Set good examples. Do not encourage them to go on crash diets, or become obsessed with weight and body image. Teens learn by example. You know their friends will go out for fast food. That does not mean you have to. Take them to the supermarket once in a while and buy good foods, go to farmer's markets, and teach them healthy eating. Don't let your kids watch you get drunk or smoke, don't expose them to habits that will harm both you and them. It may not be immediately apparent, but they do learn and will follow your example. Being a parent should mean you are an adult and carry the responsibility of childrearing seriously.

Group 2: Adult Symptoms

Age Group: Mid-20s to 30s

Remember Marcia with the postpartum depression? Marcia stopped cooking for her family after she had her baby. As her depression worsened, so did her eating habits. Marcia ate one meal a day, if that. Between caring for the baby and feeling constantly exhausted, she spent her days fatigued and dragging. No wonder: her main meal after usually skipping breakfast and lunch consisted of cereal, fast food, or a frozen dinner. There was no nutritional value in what she ate. She ate infrequently and the food she did eat was toxic to her system. Between the rapid drop in hormones (the normal aftermath of childbirth), and the lack of substantial nutrition, Marcia spent her life on the sugar roller coaster, her insulin levels either sky-high or dangerously low, counterbalanced by her blood sugar levels in constant flux. With this type of diet, she was adding insult to injury to her already stressed system.

Once we helped her balance her hormones with the supplemental progesterone, she was able to follow The Hormone Friendly Diet and we watched Marcia improve her eating habits. She liked eggs so she started having egg sandwiches on whole grain toast for breakfast. Lunch was a little trickier, but within a few weeks' time she started to eat tuna or chicken salad. Dinner became family time and Marcia started to cook: meat, or fish, along with vegetables and salad. Her husband, who was used to grabbing a slice of pizza on his way home from work, happily switched to the home-cooked meal Marcia now prepared almost every night. As her diet improved, her mood improved and finally Marcia and her husband started going out on dates. Marcia's life was now better than before she had the baby.

While most 20- and 30-year-olds do not focus on their hormones or their diets this is a great time to start making connections that will help improve life across the decades to follow.

An Aside About Alcohol in Your 20s and 30s.

Partying is an important part of the social scene of young people. While the young person's liver may easily detoxify alcohol, the rest of the body can't. Sleep, brain function, and ability to concentrate are directly impaired by excessive alcohol intake. The capacity to make hormones is significantly disrupted by the presence of alcohol in the system. Our culture encourages drinking too much and discourages and even ostracizes those who choose to drink in moderation or skip it altogether. Just because others do it, doesn't mean you must follow. I suggest practicing moderation. Enjoy life, but keep in perspective how alcohol affects you, your body and your decisions. It's not true that people are more fun when drunk. They are most fun when healthy.

Unprocessed foods high in protein (fish, fowl) and fiber (dark leafy vegetables, salads, fruit, seeds and nuts) should be the mainstay of everyone's diet.

If work or other commitments interfere, I recommend balance. If you are eating too much fast food during the week, make a point of eating lots of vegetables and unprocessed meats on the weekend. When in doubt, head for the green leafy, dark-colored foods. They are rich in nutrients and add health to your life.

GROUP 3 and GROUP 4: Premenopause and Perimenopause

Age Group: 35–55

Olga, the 35-year-old with bloating, PMS, weight gain, fatigue, and sore breasts belongs to this group. Besides needing bioidentical/human identical hormones, Olga needed some nutritional guidance too. While a teen or 20-year-old can get away with an inconsistent and not so clean diet, as we age, the situation changes dramatically. Our hormone production diminishes and it becomes imperative to take our food intake seriously. The best way to prepare for the time when hormones start to leave is to start following a healthy diet from the time we are teenagers. But if this has not been the case for you, it's never too late to improve your eating habits.

Olga never ate regular meals. She skipped breakfast, drank lots of coffee, had lunch on the run between jobs and kids. She prided herself that dinner was a family affair and she and her children ate together at least three times a week. What they had for dinner was another story. Olga prepared pasta or potatoes or rice with steak and an occasional salad. She proudly informed me that the steak was always grade A quality and low in fat. For dessert, Olga's daughter baked brownies or chocolate chip cookies. This feast might have been okay for a 20-year-old once a week, but for Olga it was a prescription for disaster.

One cannot overstate the damaging effects of fluctuating sugar and insulin levels on the body. With Olga's hormones all over the map, her diet provided fertile ground for worse hormone problems. My advice to Olga was simple. Start eating small meals every 3 to 4 hours to keep your sugar level even and minimize insulin spikes. Make your meals high in protein (egg whites, beans, fish, chicken, turkey, white unprocessed meats, nuts, soy), fiber (vegetables, seeds, nuts, fruit in small portions, mostly berries, oat, bran, quinoa, spelt, flax, wheat berries, and so forth) and limit the intake of saturated fats, starches and sugars (pasta, rice, potato, bread, muffins, bagels, cookies, cake, ice cream, and so on). Minimize the size of your evening meal, so you can digest it fast and get to sleep easily. Soups are great for the evening meal. The body digests them fast. Limit to one cup of caffeinated coffee in the morning only. Beyond its stimulatory effects on the nervous system, caffeine increases breast tenderness and cyst formation. It has also been linked to infertility and osteoporosis. Do not gamble thinking its negative effects won't affect you.

Finally, Olga started drinking water. Olga, who didn't think drinking water had any value, was shocked at the remarkable improvement in the quality of her skin once she started drinking six glasses of water a day.

Natural/human identical hormone supplementation made Olga's change in diet easier to implement, because it decreased her sugar cravings. And the change in diet improved the effectiveness of the hormones, returning Olga to a younger, more vibrant self.

For the large number of women who belong in this category, my advice is to evaluate your diet openly and objectively, make the changes necessary to feel better as early as possible and do not deviate from your course too often. If you do, gently slide back to the middle of the road and enjoy the improvement—it is highly significant.

GROUP 5: Menopause and Postmenopause

Age Group: 55-plus

Donna, a 57-year-old with a family history of osteoporosis, and Sophie, a 78-year old retired nurse, are examples of women in need of natural/bioidentical/human identical hormones who clearly understood the importance of diet in their lives. They both ate balanced meals, high protein and fiber, and limited carbohydrates and fats. They stayed away from processed meats and fast foods. They understood the value of good nutrition. They were in the group most likely to integrate proper nutrition into a healthy lifestyle. However, they also needed vitamins and supplements to further help them against the damaging effects of aging.

Supplements

My advice, although not always the same for every age group, is to supplement the diet with the following basic vitamins and supplements:

- ▶ Vitamin D—5,000 IU a day. An antioxidant, this vitamin protects against cancer, decreases the risk of heart disease and stroke and improves memory along with its highly significant role in bone formation and maintenance.

▶ Vitamin C—1,000 mg a day. An antioxidant, this vitamin stimulates immune function, helps iron absorption, protects from recurrent urinary tract infections and decreases the risk of atherosclerosis and stroke. And let's not forget, Linus Pauling won a Nobel Prize for discovering its amazing importance and lived well into his 90s taking more than 20 grams daily.

▶ Folic acid—400 mcg-1 mg a day. Decreases fibrocystic breasts, relieves PMS, decreases risk of colon cancer, and lowers homocysteine levels, which are markers of inflammation and increased risk of cardiovascular disease.

▶ Vitamin B_6—100 mg a day, and Vitamin B_{12}—100 mcg a day. Relieves hot flashes, PMS, mood swings and muscle cramps.

▶ Calcium— 500 mg a day preferably in the evening. May help build bones, decrease risk of colon cancer and stroke, and maintain normal blood pressure. Along with the other supplements it may also help relieve PMS symptoms.

▶ Magnesium—400-600 mg a day with calcium. Relieves PMS, fatigue, helps build bones, decreases angina and palpitations, is a great muscle relaxant, decreases incidence of depression, and improves intestinal regularity.

▶ Zinc—25 mg a day with calcium. Protects against dementia and depression and is an immune booster.

▶ Coenzyme Q—200 mg a day. The most potent antioxidant present in every cell in our body, it revitalizes the heart, stimulates energy production in the mitochondria at the cellular level, and delays brain aging.

▶ L-Carnitine—500–1,000 mg a day. A nonessential amino acid crucial to hormone and energy production in the mitochondria. It protects against blood clots, controls lipid levels, helps burn fat, strengthens cell membranes, and helps red blood cell production.

▶ L-Glutamine—500 mg before meals. An amino acid that stabilizes blood sugar levels and prevents insulin spikes. It works in conjunction with calcium to curb sugar cravings.

▶ Omega-3, omega-6 fatty acids—DHA and EPA, 2,000 mg/day. Antioxidants, unsaturated fatty acids, they are protectors of cell membranes and help with brain, skin, hair, joints, and immune function.

▶ Probiotics—Healthy gut bacteria immune boosters, enhancers of nutrient absorption, and supporters of intestinal flora.

▶ Digestive enzymes—Before meals to help provide enzymatic support for food digestion and breakdown of food stuffs into usable molecules.

▶ Lactoferrin (Defense)—Immune booster, protects against viruses and reduces duration of colds and flu. In my office, we use Defense, our own brand of lactoferrin to help prevent and shorten colds and flu and protect from acquiring viral infections during travel.

Before taking these supplements and vitamins consult with your physician. Interaction with medications always occurs and your physician must know what supplements you are taking and why. I stress the importance of sharing this information with your physician because achieving balanced health is a team effort and cooperation among your health care providers will improve your outcome significantly.

Finally, on the topic of supplements, please visit www.eshealth. com and read about the supplement line we've developed and work with successfully in our practice. Consider using them. Learn what combinations we use to improve hormone balance, raise energy levels, eliminate fatigue, support immune function and decrease inflammation.

Exercise

My mantra is: "Exercise should not be a source of more stress in our lives. *Intentional movement* is what is crucial to great health."

Although we are constantly bombarded with information on the importance of exercise we miss the point that exercise is yet another highly personal enterprise. Not everyone can or will get off the couch and join a spinning class three times a week.

Whether you are 20 or 70, no exercise program will work for you unless you have body awareness and treat your body with utmost respect. Before you even consider getting involved in an exercise program, you must evaluate your reasons for considering the program.

Let's say you're overweight. Depending on your age, your body configuration, state of health, genetic makeup and personality a large array of exercise options are available to you. Figuring out what fits your goals is half the battle. Staying on the program comes naturally if you see results within a reasonable period of time and if you don't perceive it as a chore. Reasonable results can usually be seen two to four months after committed and consistent adherence to a particular program. Just like everywhere else in life, there are no shortcuts to exercise.

If you are serious about implementing significant change in your physical well-being and looks, the first step is to get educated. I promise you this approach will save you money and heartache, not to mention avoid accidents. To learn about appropriate options and discover what works best for you, consult an expert in exercise physiology, a physical therapist or an experienced trainer at a well-respected gym. Make sure the person is the right one for you. If you are in your 50s don't start working out with a 20-year-old unless you are in great shape. Be reasonable in your expectations and you will see great results. Once you know how much activity you need to lose weight and/or get fit, you can find the right program and then tweak it to suit your personal needs.

Don't buy the newest exercise fad video or attempt to follow routines described in magazines. They may not be right for you, cause you to get injured and I guarantee your enthusiasm will fade faster than I can write this sentence.

Melanie is a perfect example. When I first saw her, she was 43 and small built. Because her weight had never been an issue, athletics weren't on her radar screen. Melanie had a family history of osteoporosis and being small-boned and not athletic, she was at high risk. That's why she came to see me. In addition to starting her on natural/bioidentical hormones (estradiol and testosterone), I advised her to start an exercise program focused on increasing her muscle strength. Although we discussed the importance of a gentle transition from no exercise to strength building, Melanie jumped right in. She bought a video promising fast results in 20 minutes a day. She did the routine on the video every day for two weeks. When I saw her, as a result of an urgent call, she had pulled a muscle in her lower back and her left shoulder was so painful, she had to stop exercising. Melanie was not only in pain, she was discouraged and ready to give up and settle into getting old and osteoporotic.

Gently, I pointed out the options Melanie had. If she gave up exercising, she would rapidly age and her bones would thin, leaving her hunched over and unable to wear heels. Instead, if she reconsidered the exercise, or as I preferred to call it in her case, intentional movement, she may feel better and certainly look great for an indefinite time. Melanie went along with the latter option. We found her a great trainer (also a patient in our practice) and started by focusing on stretching before the actual strength training, allowing recovery time between workouts, and varying the types of exercises. Weights, TRX bands, Pilates, and yoga together with interval and voilà, we created a program that worked for Melanie. You should see her arms now; she only wears sleeveless tops and her bone density is excellent to boot.

Genetics, Age, and Type of Exercise

Before jumping on the bandwagon of exercise, let's take a moment to evaluate some key variables that directly affect chances for success.

If ignored, genetics will create a major stumbling block. I feel badly for women who tell me that no matter how hard they exercise they can't lose weight. When I ask them about their family history, their mothers and sisters often have weight problems too. The adage "genes rule" is most relevant when developing expectations from an exercise program. If you are 5 feet tall and weigh 140 pounds and are size 12, you will never be 5 feet 10 inches tall, weigh 125 pounds and a size 2. While the shape of your body can be altered with plastic surgery (liposuction, implants, augmentations) bone structure and tendencies toward weight gain in particular areas (hips, thighs, bottom, love handles) are genetically set. So even if you do decide to get help from knife or laser, genetics will fight you and return your body to its genetically predisposed shape in no time. This knowledge should not be a deterrent from exercise or a little nip and tuck; it is meant to only help you create reasonable expectations and put things into perspective. Make the best of what you have. Don't set yourself up for failure by trying to accomplish more than humanly possible.

Which brings me to the next issue: your age. Although more people in their 60s, 70s, 80s, and on exercise on a regular basis, the type of exercise and results are different from what a younger person would obtain under the same circumstances. I marvel at the middle-age men I see who are fighting a constant uphill battle at the gym pumping iron next to buff 20-year-olds. The older guys are pulling muscles, tearing ligaments, feeling worse with each routine, and blaming themselves for being inadequate, while never addressing their age or the lack of hormones as culprits. I realize they believe that admitting getting older translates into giving up, but it certainly doesn't have to. It's most important to protect yourself from injuries that will only slow you down and make you age faster. Once you understand that aging changes your body's response to exercise, you can do exercise routines that help you stay limber and strong indefinitely.

Be gentle to yourself and you will find that even if you are 80, you can still be in good shape. Start slowly. Stretching becomes a most important part of any exercise program as we age regardless of what you read to the contrary. People who stretch on a regular basis, for a minimum of 10 minutes before and after any physical activity (intentional movement) are able to perform at the same level as people 20 years their juniors. Warming up takes longer with age, but once the joints and muscles have been lubricated and go into gear, I'll put a 60-year-old against a 40-year-old and watch out.

All too often I meet women in their 60s who are reluctant to start exercising because they never did it before and think they are too old. I believe you start and keep exercising from the moment you are born, but I also believe you can start at any age. It's never too late to start exercising; just remember Melanie's experience, pace yourself.

The type of exercise you choose is very important. Look at exercise as an investment in your future. If you think long-term you realize the more variety you bring into your life, the earlier you start, the more likely you are to stay fit as the years pile on.

My mother died at 86 of natural causes. She was old, had beaten breast cancer five years earlier, and was tired. Remarkably, though, until the last month of her life she was an avid *planned intentional movement fan*. When she was in her 60s she biked, when she was in her 70s and early 80s she took up swimming and water exercises;

even in her 80s she still moved. She was never an athlete, yet she constantly did something physical. Whether she planted flowers, walked up and down the street to say hello to her neighbors, or just did her daily sit-up and weight routine, she never stopped moving. When she was in her late 70s she moved into an assisted living complex. She quickly started a program for her neighbors that got many of them off the couch, away from the television sets, and out and about walking around the grounds every day. My mother may have been a bit ahead of her time in her commitment to preserving her ability to move and stay flexible and strong, but she certainly was successful and taught me well. Watching her over the years, I learned about the need to change exercises with advancing age. To this day, when prescribing exercise programs for my patients I always remember her example.

While it's great to join a team and become involved in track, field, and serious weight training in your teens and 20s, you must change in your 30s and 40s to more cardio-focused exercises. Staying in great shape does not mean you have to be a jock forever. Preparation starts in your teens, but persistent, consistent and age-appropriate exercise will keep you active and vital indefinitely.

The highlights of a successful approach to exercising for our general patient groups according to age are summarized in the following paragraphs. Find your group and use the guidelines, but realize that the earlier you start and the more individualized your program, the more successful you'll be.

Group 1

Age Group: Teens and Early 20s

Our American educational system includes organized physical activity. Every high school student takes mandatory physical education weekly and many participate in team sports. This is a great start. I advise parents to help their children stay focused and involved in team sports for as long as possible. Research has shown that children who stay involved in team sports through college are more disciplined, deal better with stress and integrate into society easier than their nonathletic counterparts. So what happens to those of us who do not go on to college on an athletic scholarship? Most young adults rapidly fall into the trap of overwork and little or no time for planned physical endeavors. The time to develop a consistent and successful exercise program and make it a permanent part of your life is during the early 20s. I know it's a hard concept to sell, especially when you are young and weight is not an issue age 30 seems far off and no one even knows what osteoporosis means. However, a physically active 20-year-old has more energy, concentrates better and fends off illness more than an inactive teen. And that is a fact.

General guidelines for the teens to 20s group that work and aren't difficult to integrate into everyday life:

▶ Engage in team sports.

▶ Try as many sports as possible. Exposure to many sports will help you stay in great shape and keep you entertained.

▶ Make exercise an integral part of your life. Don't let a day go by without including some type of physical activity. This is the time in life when you are building the foundation for later years. The same way you go to school to prepare for the future, create a track record of always being physically active and fit.

Group 2 and Group 3

Age Group: Late 20s to 40s

This is the group where most women have children, raising them and/or working full-time. Exercise falters as a priority. The hormone changes during these critical decades cause less damage if exercise is already a constant in our lives. Make time to exercise.

As your body changes from childbirth, lifestyle, diet and stress, your exercise program should adjust too. Time taken to exercise at this point in life represents a long-term investment in your health. This is the time to formalize an all-inclusive program of aerobic, weight/strength, flexibility and cardio fitness. If you do it right and do it now, you will stay fit for the rest of your life.

Here are basic guidelines for all to follow:

▶ Join a gym and take an aerobics class three times a week.

▶ Walk half an hour every day carrying light weights (1 to 5 lbs.).

▶ Use exercise time to socialize. Play tennis, swim, hike, mountain climb, kayak, bike, participate in a team sport. Instead of going out to lunch or for coffee, socialize while doing something physical. Learn from men; they socialize golfing, playing basketball, sailing, playing squash. You can do it too with dance classes, Zumba, Pilates, yoga, jogging, and so on.

▶ Start and stay on a daily routine of strength building and stretching. At this point in life, you can build muscles easily and starting with 3- to 5-lb weights, results can be obtained in 6 to 8 weeks of consistent exercise. Repetitions of 10 every other morning for 10 minutes before getting into the shower should become routine. Do ten women's pushups every morning. Everyone has 10 minutes to invest in their health. Just think of it like brushing your teeth.

▶ By 30, stop high-impact aerobics and NO JUMPING JACKS. They increase wear and tear on your joints and precipitate and worsen prolapses of the uterus and bladder. You may not think it applies to you now, but the dribbles when you laugh and cough of the mid-50s start right here in your 30s from too many jumping jacks and high-impact aerobics.

▶ Start taking yoga once a week. Learn to incorporate relaxation and flexibility in your exercise routine. This is the time in life when learning how to deal with stress becomes critical. Properly employed relaxation techniques preserve your health and protect your body from injuries.

▶ Learn to meditate. Guided meditation 10 minutes a day is a great start. Try www.headspace.com. Not everyone becomes a transcendental meditation expert but we can all learn to stop and take a breath and be quiet and alone for 10 minutes a day.

▶ Have a massage. Try shiatzu, deep tissue, musculoskeletal release, or lymphatic drainage. A good massage improves your flexibility, removes muscle spasms, drains excess water from your body, and protects from injuries. When choosing a massage therapist please be careful. Get information on their training and experience. Do not turn your body over to an inexperienced person who can easily, albeit unintentionally, hurt you. If you had a massage and feel worse after it, do not go to the same person again. The rule of thumb must always be: "feel better or reconsider."

▶ Dance. Take ballet, line, ballroom, tango, salsa, *any* dancing. It is a social sport good for your body and mind. "Dancing with the Stars" has put dancing into our lives so follow their example and dance!

Group 4 and Group 5

Age Group: Late 40s and Later

If you spent your whole life exercising regularly, this time is another stage in the continuum of physical activity. However, most of us are human and spend most of our youth taking our bodies for granted. Rest assured, it is never too late to start moving. It is also never too late to reap the incredible benefits of an *integrated program*. By that

I mean *hormones, supplements, diet, sleep, stress management, and exercise* working together to provide optimum vitality and health.

Natural/bioidentical/human identical hormones will turn back the clock and give your body its second chance at staying young: take advantage of this opportunity and create a bulwark against osteoporosis, heart disease and debilitating chronic illnesses. Establish an *intentional movement* routine that includes weight/resistance training, cardio, stretching and flexibility exercises.

Clark came to see me at the age of 75. He looked 20 years younger and was an avid skier and tennis player. He wanted testosterone because his sex life had started to slow and he refused to give it up. Clark's blood tests showed low testosterone levels. Six months into the therapy with testosterone Clark was doing very well. He even noticed improvement in his exercise endurance and muscle building. He felt rejuvenated and offered praise to our program. Then, one day he called to tell me, he had pulled a muscle while skiing. A week later, back on the slopes he tore a ligament. Speaking with Clark at length, he told me he felt 40 again. Because he was doing so well on the testosterone, he started to skip warm-ups and cooldowns as part of his exercise routines. And he got injured.

The key to exercise in later years is patience, body awareness and reasonable expectations. If you take your time and warm up, stretch, and limber up before and after workouts, do it consistently and listen to your body, you can do as much if not more than when you were younger. Once Clark realized that he would be protecting himself and accomplishing more by taking his time, he did not get injured again and to this day is still skiing down the slopes with the 40-year-olds. Only difference, he takes half an hour to warm up before joining his younger pals and he doesn't allow himself to get cold on the slopes, keeping his muscles and ligaments warm and well-stretched.

Here are tips for approaching exercise in our 50s to 90s, ensuring success and avoiding injuries.

▶ Before starting the day stretch for 20 minutes. Get out of bed, get on the floor, and stretch. Do sit-ups, crunches, push-ups, arm raises, and weights (2 to 4 lbs.) It doesn't matter how many; it matters that you do the entire 20 minutes.

▶ Walk every day. The more you walk the better you'll feel. Two miles is the minimum. Track your walking and make sure you hit 6,000 steps a day.

▶ Take a Pilates class. Join other women your age and get involved in gentle strengthening exercise routines with the goal of stretching you and building your flexibility. Aerobic exercise with high impact is harmful at 60. Interval training is the best for this age group. See how much better you feel and how quickly you drop extra pounds with interval training.

▶ Swim. Swimming is a great exercise. No pressure is applied to your joints and muscles become strong. And don't forget, use a swim cap to keep your hair the color you like unless you like it green.

▶ Dance. Socializing and athletic endeavors work hand in hand. You won't get old if you are physically and socially active. So combine them.

▶ Get on a treadmill whenever possible and walk at 3.5 miles an hour and an incline of 2 percent for 20 minutes. It will keep your arteries clear and give you the cardio-aerobic exercise you really need. Try a total of 30 minutes divided in 5-minute segments at 3.5 to 4 mph, alternating with 1 minute at 5 mph and if you can't do 20 minutes at once, do 10 minutes twice a day.

▶ Bike, trek, hike, canoe, ski, play tennis, ice-skate, roller-blade. Do everything you did at 40. Just warm up before and stretch after.

In the final analysis, the exercise program you undertake must be reasonable. Exercise should not be a drain or a chore, it should add to your sense of well-being, improve your mood and have you look forward to it. Exercise should not be just relegated to a means to the goal of losing weight. If you understand and heed the importance of exercise as a most important ingredient to keeping you healthy, you won't need to do it to lose weight.

Your health depends on your moving. I tell my patients all the time: "You don't need to change into workout clothes or go to a gym to get the physical activity your body craves. The opportunity to exercise exists every minute of your life so just do it."

- When you are driving your car, tighten your butt. Repeat it 10 times every 30 minutes you are in the car.
- Bring a 3-pound dumbbell to work and pump it 10 times a few times a day. Grab a water bottle, use it to pump it 10 times, then drink from it.
- When you get up in the morning, get on the floor and do 20 sit-ups before you take your shower.
- Park your car at the farthest point in the parking lot and walk to your destination.
- Don't take elevators. Just walk even if it is on the fifth floor.

Vigor and energy are directly related to the amount of movement you include in your life. And as you get older, strength and flexibility become more important. If you have strong muscles you don't get osteoporosis, regardless of your genetic make-up.

Lifestyle

We live in a stressful world. To deny it is to add more stress and lie to ourselves.

Learning to identify our stressors and then dealing with them is more reasonable and honest.

Natural/bioidentical/human identical hormones are crucial to balancing your hormones, but they cannot work optimally in a vacuum. No treatment can work if your lifestyle is counterproductive and destructive to your body and mind.

Linda was a 47-year-old nurse. She was quite knowledgeable about hormones and when she started experiencing symptoms of hormone deficiency, she came to see me. After her work-up I started her on micronized progesterone and estradiol in a cycled protocol. I saw her once a month for two months. She did not feel better. Her hot flashes diminished and her night sweats were almost gone, but overall Linda was not great. I went over her diet and exercise regimens very carefully. She was nothing short of perfect. At my wit's end, I asked her to talk to me in detail about her personal life. It turned out Linda was in trouble.

A 10-year relationship with a man had ended abruptly a few weeks before her hormone troubles started. She was embarrassed to tell her friends, co-workers, and family because they all expected her to get married and his departure was totally unexpected. Her self-confidence bottomed out.

So, she hid. She made excuses and stayed home. The stress in Linda's life was mounting. She saw no way out. No wonder the hormones weren't helping her! She went into therapy, which helped her see herself in a more forgiving light. A couple of months later, Linda started telling everyone the truth and miraculously her symptoms started to improve and the hormones worked.

Very often complaints that bring symptoms of hormone imbalance to the surface and even throw women into menopause are precipitated by major life changes. To ensure success of a treatment plan, you cannot ignore your life or think some areas are separate and should not be included in the analysis of the entire situation. Don't think your life is compartmentalized and mind and body are separate. Everything you do affects how you feel as a whole.

De-Stress

Unrelenting stress is the greatest energy zapper, and a large impediment to the successful treatment of medical and mental conditions. Regardless of thousands of studies debating the connection between stress and outcome, I can assure you from my four decades of medical experience that people who know how to deal with stress, not just superficially, but deeply and honestly, fare best in any medical situation.

A comprehensive prescription for success must include learning to de-stress. That's easier said than done. Everything we do stresses our systems. Whether it is mental stress from family issues, personal drama, work-related challenges, or physical stress in terms of eating, rest, sleep deprivation, and exercise patterns, the result is wear and tear on our entire system.

This wear and tear cannot be completely eliminated, but it can be delayed and its impact minimized.

Hormone balance plays an enormous role in our ability to tolerate stress. But even when that balance has been achieved, we must identify the stressors to which we are particularly vulnerable as individuals and figure out what can reasonably be done about them.

When you feel under significant pressure, get a diary and write. Even if it takes a few weeks or months, you will eventually pinpoint the events that precipitated the stressful feelings.

My young women patients find out very quickly that before they get their periods they feel stressed. School, work, family ties become overwhelming, difficult to handle, and they feel ready to snap.

While progesterone cream certainly abates some of the irritability, dealing with the reality of the difficulties of being a teen still exists and must be dealt with. The same thing goes for the 47-year-olds who suddenly realize they suddenly are having difficulty juggling work, family, and friends. Hormones help, but dealing with the problems and making them less stressful is an absolute must.

Stress Solutions

▶ Put the stressor in an imaginary drawer and shut it! We are accustomed to believing we must work out every problem, struggling with it until we find a solution. Some problems do not have solutions, at least for a while and rather than stressing yourself when there is no answer to be found, give yourself a break and move on.

▶ Take a deep breath out! A good friend of mine once gave me a great tape by an eastern master. I listened to it a few times. I knew I would never become a yogi, but I learned an important piece of advice from the tape. When I feel overwhelmed, I stop and take a deep breathe *out*! Somehow when you breathe in, you are bringing into your body all the stress and worry from the outside world. When you breathe out, all the stuff you held in just dissipates from you. It may not make my problems go away, but my load becomes much lighter. Try it. Take three breaths in through your nose into your lungs and belly, counting to five. Hold for the count of five and let them out through your mouth to the count of seven. See how you feel.

▶ Pause, even for a second! In tennis, the difference between an average and a good tennis player is timing. A split-second delay allows you to focus better and see where the ball is going, how to better hit it and how to direct your shot. Take the split-second delay concept and apply it to your life. Before reacting in a stressful situation, after you take a deep breath out, stop for a few seconds. In these few seconds, you can consider if it is worth reacting or if there are better ways to deal with the situation. The split-second delay allows you to become aware of yourself and your surroundings. The message is: don't react immediately because you may not need to react at all. I'm not recommending you start intellectualizing everything and lose the spontaneity that makes you unique and life interesting; just stop for a split-second, and think about what you really want to do. As we age we learn that drama is a bad thing in our lives. It creates negative energy and stress, which release cortisol and other destructive hormones. So less drama, less stress, better health.

▶ Stop feeling stuck in the past! Linda's story is a perfect example of this situation. When something happens that you have no control over, let go of it! Be sad, mourn the situation, the person, but holding on to it or trying to make believe it did not happen or wishing it hadn't happened will only make your stress levels go up. I find many male patients stuck in their youth. They believe their best days are behind them—high school football, college swimming, their 20s. If you believe the best is in your past, then that will be true. Instead, look at how you can make the present better. Don't miss today by wasting precious energy on yesterday.

▶ Take one step at a time! I think my life is overwhelming most of the time because I find myself biting off more than I can chew. I don't know how to say no. Unfortunately, I found out the hard way that if I do less, I accomplish more and leave a lot less disappointment behind. Start saying no once in a while. You'll stay focused and move ahead faster. Give up on doing 20 things at once. Think of your life as a stove. Move everything you don't need to do today to the back burner. See how much better and less cluttered your life becomes.

▶ Communicate! Clearing up misunderstandings is probably one of the least addressed lifestyle issues. We are all
so afraid of confrontation, of being perceived as a bully, of
being wrong, of being at fault and not living up to someone
else's expectations, we allow miscommunications to ruin
our lives. Do you find yourself in the same discussions
and arguments over and over again with certain people
in your life? Do you leave meetings and conversations
feeling you were not heard or understood? How often do
you wonder what the other person you were talking to was
trying to say? Poor communications skills are at the root
of so many problems in health and in life in general. Often
when people talk they Parallel Talk or Ping-Pong. People
are so busy preparing their answer and wanting to get their
point across they don't listen. The result is a stressed and
frustrated human on both sides of the conversation. And
let's not forget that we are communicating less and less
the more we just text, e-mail, Instagram, X-box, and spend
time glued to the TV set. Our social media lives divided
among Facebook, Twitter, LinkedIn, and YouTube only
serve to disconnect us from each other, eliminating the
entire concept of intimacy, nonsexual communication,
which, by the way, we never mastered enough to move
on to the present state of noncommunication anyway.
So, don't waste precious energy, take the time to listen
and relax enough to allow another point of view to filter
through. The result is you will be carrying less on your
shoulders and the world will be an easier place to be in.

▶ Have reasonable expectations! When patients come to see
me for the first time I always wonder what their expectations are. It's a very important barometer of the type of
person I am dealing with and a strong indicator of how
they will respond to my suggestions. The one extreme

is the woman who wants to walk out of the office with hormone creams in hand (even though they have to be prepared in a lab away from the office or picked up at the pharmacy) and start treatment immediately. The other extreme is the woman who, after spending time and money on an extensive consultation with me, laboratory testing, specific formulations of hormones, and extensively reading educational materials, spends months thinking about when and how to start the new regimen. Fortunately for all, most people fit somewhere in the middle. For those extremists, I fear they will be disappointed because their expectations are not reasonable. Be realistic. I tell my new hormone patients: let's give it three months. Let's balance, tweak doses and formulations of hormones, and talk about it once a month or more often if necessary. Begin with the premise that it will take three months to get to a decent balance. I know most people take less, but I allow us some wiggle room. This way I don't feel overly pressured and the patients are invariably pleasantly surprised. In times of transition, like perimenopause to menopause and some-times during change of seasons or during times of stress, hormones need to be adjusted and carefully titrated. The same is true for the rest of your life. As long we are alive we change and change needs to be addressed gently and kindly.

▶ Get a new attitude! The most important de-stressor may simply be changing your outlook. Take the attitude that your life is as good as it will ever be. Rather than always looking to improve the future or blaming yourself for the past, learn to treat yourself kindly now, in this moment. I'm not referring to getting the obligatory manicure, the massage and facial or the trip to the mall, I mean some-thing simpler. Give yourself permission to be you, to be who you really are. Give yourself permission to age, but not to give into disease or frailty. If you are 50, don't try to be 30, just be the best 50-year old you could be for you. Don't use anyone else's standards: define yourself as the unique person you are. Take responsibility for your life and either accept it as it is or change it for the better with your new attitude.

▶ Engage! I get very nervous when I see aging women who are depressed. Hormones will make them feel better, but to what end? The kids grown, the husband not present (emotionally or physically), women who are isolated are at risk. Boredom is a dangerous place to find yourself when you are past your 30s. Get out of the house, join a club, a church, a charity, or just get a job. Boredom is a place we go to hide from our feelings and our problems. Your mind knows that if you address the reality of your situation you have to do something about it, so it shuts down. Don't let it! Keep a diary and see what is really going on in your mind and in your heart. The entries will show you where you are and if you are hiding from troublesome reality issues.

▶ Retirement is a danger spot for most active people. Andrew, a construction worker patient of mine, became more and more of a couch potato over a period of six months after his retirement. His wife brought him to me for testosterone supplementation because she thought he was depressed. Testosterone improved his libido, but did not get him off the couch. I suggested he start walking every day. He said his arthritis was bothering him too much. I suggested he go to church with his wife on Sunday. He didn't. The service conflicted with his favorite Sunday morning news show. I told him to tape the show and just go to church. He reluctantly agreed. The minister must have heard my prayers because he asked Andrew to help supervise a construction project at the church. Andrew got off the couch, went back to work, and even walked the two miles to church and bought a treadmill for his basement. See what a little engaging can do? Don't think you cannot find the little place that opens the door to your getting back into the world as a participant.

▶ Sleep! We have addressed the relationship between sleep disorders and hormone imbalance in Chapter 3, but I want to reinforce its significance. Sleep is sacred. If you don't get it, you get cranky, your focus is off, you are fatigued, you walk in a fog, your brain and body don't function optimally, you get sick, and your hormones become confused and out of sync. Sleep is so crucial for hormone production it cannot be overstated. When hormones are in balance and we can sleep, we must ensure that other factors do not deter us from sleeping, because sleep equals youth. You sleep well = you stay healthier longer and certainly look better.

Here are some tips to help improve your chances for a good night's sleep with the understanding that your hormones are in good balance as a first and most necessary step to getting the sleep you need:

▶ Clear your bedroom of things that don't belong there. All work-related stuff must go. Close the shades, keep the room cozy, cool, and uncluttered.

▶ Eliminate the TV. Either remove the TV set from your bedroom or just make sure it is off when you go to sleep. Do not leave the TV on. The sounds and light from it will continue to enter your brain and the quality of your sleep will be diminished. Television is the single most common deterrent to sound sleep. It keeps us from getting into

REM sleep, the deep renewing and revitalizing type of sleep we all desperately need.

▶ Watch the timing of your last meal. Eating a heavy dinner late will interfere with good sleep. Go to sleep lighter, you'll sleep better. Alcohol does not help with better sleep quality. It may help you fall asleep faster, but it will wake you up earlier and your sleep will be restless and unsatisfying and the dehydration and toxicity alcohol brings to your body will interfere with the beneficial aspects of sleep.

▶ Don't exercise too close to bedtime. Those wonderful hormones that make us feel good, endorphins, when we exercise are also going to stop us from getting the deep sleep we need to renew ourselves. To unwind do not exercise within two hours of going to sleep.

And for my final advice: a little improvement, one little step at a time, will change your whole life for the better in no time.

Be nice to yourself. You are unique; celebrate your uniqueness, don't hide it or bury it in trying to be like everybody else.

If you are tired, sleep. Things will wait. If you are sad, cry. You'll feel better.

When you are happy, enjoy it. Others will enjoy it with you.

CHAPTER 11

What About Men?

Martha, a patient and a friend who is 48, got married last year. She found the right guy.

He adores her, she worships him, they have fun together, and they cope well with all the kids and exes in their lives. Martha tells me that Mark is very loving and she's never been happier. She is on bioidentical hormones, supplements, and The Hormone Friendly diet along with exercise and she's going through menopausal changes without problems. However, Mark seems to be having some trouble. At times, Mark's mind says "yes" but his body isn't listening; his moods are erratic and his erections are flagging. They tried Viagra, which helped as long as he didn't eat fatty meals and they also know that impotence is only a reflection of the state of his vascular system in general. Martha doesn't want Mark to have a heart attack, she doesn't like medication in his body to mask what may be more trouble than the issue with erection. It took too long to find him and she doesn't want to lose him.

His erection problem isn't the only concern. His once buff body isn't so buff any more. He does go to the gym, still pumps iron, he always looked great, but at 50, something has changed—he's getting a little soft in the middle and he's even getting a little beer belly. He thought this was just part of aging. Everyone gets this way in their 40s and 50s after all. Then he read an article about the increasing use of testosterone supplementation in middle-aged men in *The New York Times Magazine* and started seeing Low-T ads on ESPN. Hopeful, he went to his doctor. Unfortunately for Mark, his doctor said he doesn't believe in information disseminated through consumer channels. He only gets his information from medical journals and the American Urologic Society and he's not comfortable with testosterone supplementation due to its potential for fueling prostate cancer. He offered to do a prostate evaluation and possible biopsy if his PSA was elevated but refused to consider testosterone and couldn't understand why Viagra or Cialis wasn't enough to make Mark happy.

Martha brought Mark to see me and after doing a thorough evaluation, bloods, reviewing stress test results from his cardiologist, and spending time with him trying to get some insight into the person he was, I started him on micronized testosterone cream. After a couple of months Mark experienced remarkable changes. He lost some of his beer belly and started to feel rejuvenated when he saw his muscles return. And Martha tells me, he's now chasing her around the house, the way he did when they first got together.

Why would men and women be different when it comes to the importance of hormones and their depletion as we age?

When I became involved with the study of hormones, I never thought in terms of men. My involvement was mostly based on personal experience and need. I wanted a safe solution for my personal symptoms of hormone deficiency and by association found solutions for my female patients. No sooner did I focus my practice on natural/bioidentical/human identical hormone supplementation for women than they started bringing their men.

When I first started practicing medicine, my knowledge about male hormones came from the education I received in medical school. That was in the 1970s and although I went to a progressive medical school, it was still a time when hormones were not a popular topic. We were taught very little more than "testosterone is the main male hormone." All we were taught was that testosterone was the hormone that differentiates men from women. It is made in the testicles and is responsible for the development of secondary sexual characteristics and the production and multiplication of sperm. Secondary sexual characteristics include a young boy's voice change, the growth of muscle and pubic hair, the typical pungent male perspiration odor, and the growth of the penis and testicles to adult size. Testosterone makes men stronger than women physically and enables them to develop beautifully sculptured bodies when following a regular workout program. And yes, testosterone is probably responsible for the way men think and process problems. That is where my basic education on testosterone ended.

What followed in my medical school course about male endocrinology was a series of syndromes and illnesses associated mostly with testosterone deficiency. Oddly enough, they all seem to occur in young men, unlike the later timing of the appearance of hormone problems in women.

Once you made it through puberty and adolescence, you brought down undescended testicles, treated the rare case of testicular cancer, an occasional inflammation or infection of the foreskin, or addressed poor sperm motility in infertile men, testosterone pretty much disappeared from the medical vocabulary. The exception was in the minimal discussion of the use of anabolic steroids by athletes trying to build huge muscle mass. It referred to the shrinkage in testicles these preparations caused and when HIV became prevalent, testosterone and HGH were used to improve cachexia (weight and muscle loss).

Testosterone Today

I rarely heard the terms male menopause or andropause until about 15 years ago. In my extensive research on hormones I never read an article decisively connecting male hormone deficiencies with symptoms at midlife. Looking back over the decades I've spent in private practice, I wonder why my profession overlooked the clear relation between men's midlife changes and hormone deficiency.

Ironically, after the publication of *The Hormone Solution* in 2002, I submitted a proposal for a book on male hormones to my publisher. The response was negative. I was told, men were not interested in reading about male hormones. I don't think they were right. Tell that to all the men lining up to get testosterone these days.

Male menopause is technically known as andropause, adult hypogonadism, or male climacteric. The reason andropause has never been in the public spotlight is because most men who experience it have been reluctant and unwilling to acknowledge its existence. This is ironic, since women to this day try to deny their own menopause more than one would think. So men and women are more alike than you might think, especially in this area.

The fact that testosterone levels drop naturally in men during middle age is little known. I don't know why it should be so surprising that men are physiologically similar to women. Just like women, when men start aging, their hormones start to decline. After the age of 40, testosterone levels drop more than 1 percent per year, thus leaving men depleted of their most important hormone by the age of 50.

Symptoms of testosterone deficiency in men present quite often, and closely resemble symptoms of hormone insufficiency in women. Middle-age gut, couch potato stance, depression, mood swings, irritability, even night sweats define the aging male. Look at the man in his 50s who is unsuccessfully trying to build muscle mass. Yes, he is aging, but it is his decreasing testosterone levels that make him ineffective when he tries to bulk up. It is not that he suddenly stopped trying.

Unfortunately, the medical profession has not been keen on addressing this obvious similarity to menopause. To male doctors andropause doesn't have a pretty ring to it; it's about aging. Men are more afraid than women to address the inevitability of this process. With men like Mick Jagger fathering children into their 70s, men like to deny that they are having the same problems as aging women. However, men who father children naturally in their 80s are as rare as women who give birth in their 50s.

As women started to openly address their issues with hormone deficiencies in the 1990s, an interesting paradox occurred. Although not immediately acknowledged as a problem, the issue of the decline in sexual performance encountered by many middle-aged men moved to a more visible position as well. Maybe not as prominently displayed in the mass media (although Low-T is certainly catching on), but nonetheless its presence started being felt in the medical community. Not that researchers haven't been studying male andropause for decades, along with the effects of reduced levels of testosterone in the aging process. It's just that the news never got to you or your doctor... pretty much like the story of hormones in women.

The Science Behind Testosterone and Male Menopause/Andropause

Sadly, the importance of testosterone in men's health has been minimized and demonized since 1939. At that time Dr. Charles Huggins, a physiologist who worked with prostate cancer, reported in a medical journal a case study of a man who had metastatic prostate cancer and high testosterone levels concomitantly. He raised the question of a connection between testosterone and prostate cancer. Huggins received a Nobel Prize in 1966 and concluded that testosterone affects PSA levels. Never again was that connection made in any medical study or report since.

Unfortunately, medicine is subject to the same rumor mill as any other profession. The story was too good to let go and testosterone became indelibly connected to prostate cancer. Dr. Huggins effectively ruined the lives of millions of men who would have benefited from more testosterone in their lives. He also helped give rise to a huge industry of men having prostate biopsies and massive surgeries, often getting rid of healthy prostates, scared just like women of breast cancer. The outcome is often a significant decrease in quality of life, leaving men impotent and incontinent, prevalent beyond what any of us would expect. In 2007, Dr. Abraham Morgentaler from Harvard reviewed the entire medical literature on proof of the connection between prostate cancer and testosterone and failed to find a study or case report to substantiate that connection.

Urologists, just like many gynecologists, still refuse to treat men with testosterone unless they have a negative prostate biopsy, in spite of science that proves that testosterone keeps men healthy and vibrant as they age and doesn't cause prostate cancer.

Study after study shows how testosterone protects the heart and bones, improves the mood and prevents frailty in aging men. And yes, testosterone does improve erections. Do men need medication to maintain their erections or do they need testosterone?

Pharmaceutical companies saw an obvious opportunity in the population of aging men with erectile dysfunction, ED. Unfortunately, the treatment addressed one isolated symptom and not the root cause of male andropause. By approaching the problem from the angle of one symptom only, the larger issue of what male menopause does can be easily sidestepped and kept in the closet.

Before the real issues associated with male menopause could even be acknowledged, the treatment for impotence flooded the market.

Viagra

Viagra came onto the market like gangbusters in February 1998. It carried a resounding message: "Our manhood is at risk, we have a problem with erections and we are going to correct it quickly before anyone gets a chance to take a closer, more in-depth look at what is really causing the problem in our aging men."

So Viagra moved into our consciousness. Practically every middle-aged patient in my practice called asking for prescriptions for Viagra. I learned about it from the media and my Pfizer pharmaceutical representative, who came calling to my office with free samples of the new magic drug. It was odd; one day there was *no* conversation about impotence, the next, it was the hottest topic from Wall Street to the kids on Main Street. Commercials for the product with politicians like Bob Dole were all over TV changing the face of impotence, henceforth called, erectile dysfunction.

Although I am very open-minded, I was hesitant to write the prescriptions. I had nothing against the quick fix Viagra promised men, but I was worried that the wrong man would take it and he would become mortally ill from it. My fear came from the understanding of how Viagra works. It increases the blood flow to the penis and the pelvic organs in general. It brings more blood to the penis and as a result, a harder erection. Great, exactly what we all want, but at what cost? What if the man is older, has high blood pressure, atherosclerosis, plaques, vascular disease, or heart failure?

Viagra, by diverting blood from the heart, lung, and brain, leads to a rapid drop in blood pressure to the organs that need the blood flow the most. This increases the risk for potential strokes and heart attacks. I didn't want to scare anyone but I discouraged older men who had atherosclerotic disease from using it. Unfortunately, the very reason for their problems with erections was because they had plaques (atherosclerosis) in the blood vessels supplying the penis to begin with. They were the men on medications for high blood pressure and cholesterol. They were also suffering from impotence, a highly disturbing side-effect of anti-hypertensive medication. A catch-22 situation: the men who need the medication the most are at highest risk of getting complications from it. And the erectile dysfunction was in fact a symptom of cardiac dysfunction anyway. So what was this all about?

Despite the dilemma of its side-effects Viagra opened a door. Its sheer existence acknowledges that men experience significant and disturbing problems as they age.

Men need help too.

Male Hormones and Sex

To feel sexual interest, you need hormones. When men go from their mid-30s onto their mid-40s they undergo significant changes. Their hormone levels, specifically testosterone, start to dwindle. Since men never talk about hot flashes and night sweats and rarely address their moods, we never knew they experience them. And when it comes to erections, women wouldn't have the heart to talk about a man having problems in that area and men would never discuss it. Testosterone made in the testicles and adrenal glands starts waning with age and, just like hormones with women, as its quality and quantity declines, symptoms start to appear.

Finally, in the past decade, testosterone supplementation has entered the conventional world of prevention, wellness, integrative medicine, functional medicine, anti-aging medicine, anything you want to call prevention. However, it has not yet moved into the mainstream of medicine or become a topic for dinner conversation the way menopause is. Although recently men have started to admit to experiencing symptoms previously reserved to women, the door is only slightly ajar. In my practice, in response to the need, I have been working with testosterone supplementation in men for almost two decades.

George is a 57-year-old retired policeman. He loves to read, tend to his garden, and play with his grandchildren. George became depressed five years ago when an injury he experienced at work forced him to retire. He saw a psychiatrist and was placed on an antidepressant. The medication never worked, but George stuck with it. His mental condition deteriorated and no matter what medication the psychiatrist added it only made matters worse. George developed severe mood swings and his sex drive disappeared. One night he saw a TV segment on testosterone on the local news. The doctor interviewed recommended the hormone for the treatment of depression in middle-aged men. I saw George shortly thereafter. His wife brought him to me because his own doctor refused to give him a prescription for testosterone. I started him on a combination of testosterone cream, supplements, and a diet and exercise program specifically aimed at improving his mood and stamina. Over a period of six months, George discontinued the use of the antidepressants and had no recurrence of depression or mood swings. Today, 11 years later, George takes testosterone injections which he gives himself twice a week in his skin along with HCG (human chorionic gonadotropin) that keep his testicles from shrinking (an occasional side-effect of injectable testosterone). He loves his regimen, his PSA and all other laboratory tests are normal, his cholesterol is low, and he doesn't take any medications.

George is typical of the men I care for in our practice.

Sidney is a large man. He weighs 235 pounds, stands 6 feet 5 inches tall, and was 65 years old when I first saw him. His wife, Lara, a petite 5-foot, 100-pound, 43-year-old, appears tiny next to her man. They came to see me together. She was going through hormone changes and he came along for moral support. They were recently married. Their sex life before the wedding was wonderful, they felt like teenagers. But soon after, something changed. Lara lost interest in sex and Sidney's sex drive took a nosedive as well. He had been a body builder, but now he was having trouble keeping his muscle mass. Needless to say, these problems caused him significant angst. I tested both of their hormone levels. While Lara's hormones were within normal limits, Sidney's testosterone was practically inexistent. His PSA, reflecting the function of his prostate gland, was normal. I started him on testosterone in the form of Androgel 1 percent, daily. Two months later their sex life returned to normal and he no longer complained about muscle building problems. Today, he is taking Androgel 1.62 percent with thyroid and supplements along with The Hormone Friendly Diet (www.eshealth.com). He lost 40 pounds and his life is exactly as he wished it to be.

Daily female patients bring up the topic of male menopause/andropause. The question invariably is "how can I help my husband/lover/partner?" The answer is clear and simple and backed by science: "supplement his testosterone." So, why aren't more doctors prescribing it? Do doctors still consider testosterone outside the area of conventional medicine? For our sake and our men's sake, I hope not. What used to be the domain of body builders and athletes is now without a doubt a normal part of any man's world. To provide the proper solutions to the men, conventional medicine must evolve.

Samuel is 54. He is a physician. He has been having problems with erections, muscle building and depression for years. He has taken his bloods hundreds of times looking for something abnormal to treat. His bloods have always been normal and his testosterone within normal limits. Unfortunately, Samuel was a conventional physician and he didn't realize that the blood tests that may have been within normal limits didn't truly reflect what was normal for Samuel. Since most men do not know what their baseline testosterone levels are at 25, we have no way of knowing if the testosterone level we check at 54 is normal for that particular man. So, we should start testing every man's testosterone level when he is young. This way we can learn what normal is for each individual and treat older men with testosterone based on information that applies to them.

Samuel understood the need for a common-sense approach in medicine but could not find a physician to tell him how much and what form of testosterone he needed. His urologist friend told him he needed a prostate biopsy even though his PSA (of questionable reliability as a diagnostic test for prostate dysfunction anyway) was low. The biopsy is a painful test and Samuel didn't want to do it. The urologist refused to give him a prescription. Three years passed until I met Samuel at a conference on anti-aging medicine. He was suffering and felt awful. Achy joints, depression, hair loss, weight gain, constant fatigue, and no libido. How can a doctor help patients when he can't find anyone to help him? We worked together to take care of him. Once on testosterone, he felt great. He found his old self again.

Before we go on, let's pause and look at the most common symptoms associated with testosterone depletion in the average, healthy man usually over 40:

▶ Inability to build muscle as easily as at age 20
▶ Problems losing weight as easily as at age 20
▶ Inability to ejaculate as often as at age 20
▶ Problems maintaining an erection as long as at age 20
▶ Diminished sex drive
▶ Depression and loss of excitement about life and career
▶ Irritability
▶ Moodiness
▶ Anger management issues
▶ Fatigue
▶ Insomnia and other sleep disorders
▶ Having to urinate at least once a night
▶ Lack of energy

Even if these symptoms aren't exactly the same as those experienced by women as a result of hormone depletion, they are eerily similar.

Just like women, certain men suffer from symptoms, incapacitating to varying degrees, while some sail through this period of their lives with minimal problems and settle into the next stage without much trouble. Those who do have difficulties are easy to identify. Just like their female counterparts, these men's lives are turned upside down. Coping mechanisms fail and the aging process becomes unmanageable.

Allen came to see me in a state of quiet desperation. He was a successful 52-year-old attorney. His life had been on an even keel. When he turned 50, things started to unravel. He stopped enjoying work, he had difficulties with relationships with family and friends, even stopped playing golf, his favorite hobby. His wife suggested he see a psychiatrist. The psychiatrist spent a long time talking to Allen, finally deciding to start him on Prozac. Allen felt a little better. He seemed to regain some of his lost *joie de vivre*, he even returned to his Saturday morning golf game.

But something still wasn't right. The psychiatrist raised the dose of Prozac, and added another antidepressant for better balance (Wellbutrin). Allen became groggy and the little sex drive he had was gone. His wife, a patient in our practice doing very well on bioidentical/human identical hormones and supplements, diet and exercise was coping well and Allen's problems worried her. One day, at work, Allen lost his temper and spun out of control. During an important meeting he started screaming and acting totally out of character. Embarrassed, he apologized and that same evening asked his wife for help. She brought him to me. First, I recommended a cardiologist do a thorough evaluation, then I tested Allen's bloods, including PSA, testosterone and the other hormone levels you know from previous chapters. His testosterone level was very low (total was 120ng/dl and free was 3.5ng/dl). He was depressed and anxious at the same time. The psychotropic medications were not helping. They were only masking the problems. After an extensive consultation I started Allen on transdermal testosterone cream which he wanted to get from a compounding pharmacy since he wasn't a fan of FDA-approved medications. We checked his blood hormone levels every six weeks for a few months. By the time his total testosterone levels neared 600, Allen felt well enough to stop taking antidepressant medications. It only took two months to get Allen back to the life he thought he'd permanently lost.

Allen's story is the rule for men in their 40s and 50s who start taking testosterone supplementation. The unfortunate exceptions are the men who don't know about the miraculous recoveries achieved through testosterone supplementation. Because they don't know about the importance of testosterone in their lives, they either ignore bothersome and destructive symptoms, or take antidepressant medications prescribed by physicians unfamiliar with the benefits and safety of the testosterone option. Just a thought: do you think there is such a thing as antidepressant deficiency? I don't. Hormone deficiency is the most likely problem in these cases and can only be resolved with proper hormone balancing.

Testosterone Testing

When I started seeing men in need of testosterone supplementation, I couldn't find any clinical guidelines in the medical literature. No recommendations for dosing or systems of administration for testosterone in healthy men looking to help prevent aging and frailty existed. Interestingly, in the fields of prevention, testosterone was first recognized as the feel-good hormone for women looking to maintain and improve their sex drive in their 40s and later years. Although testosterone is *the* male hormone, little is reported on its use in men for similar purposes, in either conventional or alternative medical literature. Rare articles in the scientific journals reflect a sense of surprise when men treated with their own hormone for impotence and depression improve on testosterone. Ironically, Dr. Charles-Édouard Brown-Séquard, a famous neurologist, reported in the 1800s injecting himself with extracts of sheep and other animal testicles and feeling strong and virile. His fellow physicians thought him mad.

In July 2000, Dr. Jay Adlersberg, health and medical reporter for New York's WABC-TV, reported that more than 4 million men in the U.S. suffer from low testosterone. He also added that low testosterone may cause "impotence, depression and fatigue." His report concluded with patient testimonials praising the remarkable results of testosterone supplementation. After six months in this particular study, the participants reported increase in lean body mass, sex drive and energy levels. Since then, many other studies followed and reinforced the positive impact of supplemental testosterone in aging men, not limited to sexual prowess, but also preventing frailty, improving cardiac function, enhancing muscle development and improving mood.

However, the road to openly treating men with testosterone by primary care physicians and urologists is still unpaved. Andropause, or male menopause, is still a rarely used word in our society. Andropause has not come out of the closet yet. As prevention becomes the newest medical specialty it is in the best position to educate physicians about andropause. Diagnosing hormone deficiencies in men requires detective work and just like with women an integrated approach to diet, exercise, lifestyle, sleep and supplements along with thyroid and more.

Administration of Testosterone Supplementation

A significant drawback to testosterone supplementation has been its method of administration. Testosterone cannot be given by mouth because it does not get absorbed from the stomach. For years, the only method in use was by injection. Most likely, this situation precluded testosterone supplementation from becoming popular with the public at large. For years, injectables were reserved for the very young or those sick with severe medical needs, not commonly used by men wanting to stay young and healthy.

A patch called Androderm was approved by the FDA in 1995. Initially it was used in men with testosterone deficiency diseases and AIDS-related malnutrition. Body builders quickly began using it and women too. Androderm did not make a big splash with middle-aged men. It wasn't marketed to the middle-aged man who needed testosterone most and the urologists wouldn't prescribe it because of the erroneous belief testosterone fueled prostate cancer.

In 2000, Androgel 1% testosterone gel came to the market. The FDA approved it for "treatment of low testosterone levels linked to decreased sex drive, impotence, reduced lean body mass, decreased bone density and lowered mood and energy levels." Androgel is a bioidentical/human identical testosterone in gel form, with good absorption. Sadly, it was also marketed to the wrong population of men.

As men started to learn about the benefits of testosterone in prevention, aging, and wellness, studies appeared to support the use and safety of testosterone. A well-known study from Australia reflected the results of an exhaustive 19-year follow-up of thousands of men between the ages of 24 and 67. Beneficial results of testosterone involved more than enhanced sexuality and muscle mass. Positive cardiac effects on the men who participated in the study were a welcome finding.

Adroderm, Androgel, Testim, and Axiron along with newer FDA-approved and compounded formulations of bioidentical/human identical testosterone are in use today and insurance companies pay for their use in wellness and disease prevention. There are also synthetic preparations of the hormone.

What About Men?

Testosterone cypionate, enanthate, and propionate are the injectable forms. They are used in twice-weekly doses under the skin or intramuscularly. Many men prefer the rapid rise in blood levels they cause and how that makes them feel. These can be obtained at any regular pharmacy, or can be individually compounded in specialized pharmacies.

In our programs, we successfully integrate individualized dosing of injectables under the skin or in the muscle testosterone with thyroid, HCG, supplements, diet, exercise, and lifestyle in a comprehensive, medically supervised, thoughtful program that treats the entire man. I strongly advise you talk to your doctor and together evaluate your particular situation. Once the diagnosis of testosterone deficiency is made, you owe it to yourself to get the best preparation for you. Work with your doctor and find the type of supplementation best suited for your symptoms and lifestyle. If your doctor is not up-to-date on the use of testosterone in prevention find a doctor who is. You don't need to suffer or be a victim and accept aging as the only alternative.

CHAPTER 12

IV Infusions

No conversation about hormones and prevention can end without discussing the use of IV infusions to improve quality of life.

Until 20 years ago, the only place you could get an IV infusion was in the hospital. IVs were reserved for the very sick. IV hydration, albeit a common-sense way to eliminate dehydration and speed up recovery from viruses or food poisoning, was not an option outside the Emergency Room.

A few doctors in alternative medicine started doing IV pushes to provide patients with supplements and vitamins.

While conventional medical training doesn't provide any education or guidance in how to deliver IV nutrients to patients in doctors' offices it certainly is a very much needed tool for prevention.

In our practice we've been using IV infusions to:

▶ improve immune function

▶ boost energy

▶ hydrate

▶ detoxify

▶ reduce inflammation

IV Infusions

▶ enhance pre and post operative function
▶ combat jet lag
▶ shorten duration of viruses

and help our patients lead the highest quality life at all times. For more on our IVs, please go to Appendix C.

Afterword

This book represents the wisdom acquired over more than 35 years of my personal clinical experience and research. It arose initially from a need to find concrete, safe and definitive solutions to my own hormone problems. As a woman and a practicing physician, I quickly realized I could not find a satisfactory solution for the overwhelming and destructive symptoms produced by hormone imbalance, using the tools my conventional training offered. When I turned to alternative options, the results were not any better. The treatments available in the area of hormone imbalance are an open sore for both conventional and alternative practitioners. Ridiculous debates over terminology have led to the deprivation of millions of men and women who don't need to suffer.

All scientists agree: hormones make up the fabric of our lives. They define us as men and women when we are young, they keep us healthy or make us sick, and yet the education we get about them is vague, contradictory, and inconsistent. Many researchers and clinicians allude to the connection between hormones and PMS, postpartum depression, mood swings, sexual dysfunction, migraines, weight gain, infertility, and even sleep disorders. Yet few take that important knowledge to the next level and learn to use human identical hormones to prevent disease and enhance wellness. Authoritative affirmation that hormones are the root cause of these symptoms, regardless of age, is present in the medical literature but it's largely ignored. Unequivocally, the scientific community knows that hormone levels change every minute of the day, so why get hung up on one or two changes: menopause or puberty? Once you make the connection that hormones are continually changing and the changes affect everything about your life, adolescence, perimenopause or menopause are a lot less scary and no longer devastating.

If I had not become sick with hot flashes and night sweats and experienced undesirable side-effects of conventional medications myself, I would not have become an expert in hormones. If I had not spent thousands of dollars on herbal remedies without experiencing relief, I would not have been motivated to search for a better solution. If I hadn't read every article in conventional medicine, leaving me feeling cheated by the lack of validity in the data, I wouldn't have done my own research. I had no option but to take it upon myself to formulate viable and lasting solutions that would not just help me but every woman and man I came across.

This connection became the first step in the sequence that led to the making of this book. I have provided you with the scientific basis and clinical proof that helped me reach the simple yet life-changing conclusions you now have access to as well.

The second step was finding the solution. But before I found the natural/bioidentical/human identical hormone solution, I had to objectively and seriously address other options available. I have introduced you to the conventional and alternative treatments I evaluated before reaching the natural/human identical hormone solution. I thought it important to share this information with you for a number of reasons. Even today many physicians you will see have no idea what natural/bioidentical hormones are. So, they will offer other options to you or dismiss your request for bioidentical hormone as an alternative snake oil. It is important for you to know what your options are, how they work and what their pitfalls are. This book is designed to help you make informed decisions. It serves to empower you and give you the strength to stand firm on your convictions. If you choose to try other options, be it conventional or alternative, I urge you to exercise caution and never become a victim in the process. If this is your first exposure to natural/bioidentical/human identical hormones, I hope you notice their actions and become your own testimonial to the miracle they are.

The decision to use natural/bioidentical/human identical hormones must arise from knowledge and strength, not desperation and fear. And finally, please don't work around your doctor when taking them. This book has given you the most up-to-date scientific information your doctor needs to feel comfortable prescribing natural/bioidentical hormones.

"Good solutions are simple solutions," a Nobel Prize-winning professor I had in medical school once taught me. This is a simple solution—nature's solution. Using natural/bioidentical/human identical hormones, I have total confidence in the information I present to you. Tens of thousands of patients and physicians I train and treat are the testimonials. Take the book to your doctor and start the program now.

APPENDICES

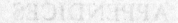

APPENDIX A

Physiology of Hormones

It all started with the most primitive of glands in our brain—the master gland, the hypothalamus.

Hormones are produced by many organs, but their production and actions are always rigidly controlled by the master gland, the hypothalamus (*hi-po-THA-la-mus*, a pinhead structure buried in the middle of the brain, above the pituitary gland). The hypothalamus literally supervises the synchronization of hormone release. We don't know how the hypothalamus got to be in charge of all hormone balance. While studied for many decades the most commonly accepted belief is that the hypothalamus is a very old organ linked to early animal evolution; allegedly there before the pituitary gland existed and before sexes were differentiated. Its role was to control basic body functions—heartbeat, breathing, digestion, reproduction, excretion. Throughout evolution, the hypothalamus has maintained its controlling role; it makes one hormone and that hormone coordinates the release or stoppage of all sex hormones: **Gonadotropin-Releasing Hormone (GnRH).**

Through a system of blood vessels inside the brain, this hormone goes directly to the pituitary and stimulates it to release its own set of hormones, with the final role of modulating production of sex hormones by the ovaries, testes, thyroid, and adrenal glands; the hormones they produce are estrogen, progesterone and testosterone. This one hormone (GnRH) monitors the production and effects of hormones made by the pituitary, thyroid, ovaries, testicles and adrenals.

Another hormone produced by the hypothalamus that is getting increasing amount of interest is oxytocin. Oxytocin was initially believed to be solely responsible for the dilation of the cervix during labor, childbirth and stimulation of the nipples to start producing milk but now more evidence has come to light connecting oxytocin to behavior. Connectivity, attachment and social associative behaviors are now correlated to increased production of oxytocin, leading to its nickname, "the love hormone." While more information will be forthcoming as more about oxytocin is studied, many are trying to bottle it already, but in conventional medicine it is all too commonly used intravenously to use induce labor. Oral oxytocin does not get absorbed and many people waste time and money buying it from compounders or the internet.

Along the evolutionary ladder, a new endocrine organ developed between the hypothalamus and other end organs (heart, lung, stomach, ovary, testicle, adrenal). That organ is the pituitary gland.

The Modern Master Gland—The Pituitary

Below the hypothalamus, buried in the middle of the brain, lies the pituitary gland. While we consider the hypothalamus a primitive, old remnant of an antique glandular system, the pituitary is much newer. It is the modern-age master gland. Arbitrarily divided by physiologists into anterior and posterior portions, the pituitary produces a lot of different hormones affecting pretty much all body functions. All sex hormone-releasing and inhibiting factors are produced by the anterior portion of the pituitary gland. It is there, in an area of a few millimeters, that the headquarters of hormone regulation are located.

The anterior pituitary is in charge of stimulating or blocking the release of the principal sex hormones: estrogen, progesterone, and testosterone. This is accomplished through the actions of two hormones secreted by the anterior pituitary: follicle-stimulating hormone (FSH) and luteinizing hormone (LH). FSH and LH are directly responsible for cycling the production of estrogen and progesterone by the organs that produce them (ovaries, adrenals and corpus luteum, the follicle left in the ovary after ovulation has taken place). FSH stimulates estrogen production, LH stimulates progesterone production. FSH and LH together balance estrogen and progesterone levels.

Another sex-related hormone produced by the pituitary, prolactin is only released after a woman gives birth. Its role is to stimulate the breast to produce milk along with the oxytocin produced by the hypothalamus, and to shrink the size of the uterus back to normal.

One more hormone of note produced by the pituitary is Thyroid Stimulating Hormone (TSH), the hormone that is the source of much confusion to both physicians and patients as far as its role in the diagnosis of thyroid function. Over the past three decades the absolute role of TSH in the diagnosis of low thyroid function has been challenged and for now the division between the old way of thinking promulgated by the American Endocrine Society and the modern thought leaders in prevention has widened to the point that many physicians and patients are choosing to disregard the test altogether in favor of symptoms and other simpler tests when making the diagnosis of low thyroid, with the goal of preventing disease.

How Do FSH and LH Work?

Let's take an average 28-day cycle, when you are not pregnant. Let's start with Day 1. You have your period. Your estrogen and progesterone levels are practically nil. The lack of hormones in your system has led you to get your period. This is a very important point to remember. When you have a period, you do not have estrogen or progesterone circulating in your system. Their drop specifically brings on periods. That is normal and natural.

GnRH from the hypothalamus and FSH from the pituitary are excreted in response to the level of estrogen circulating in your bloodstream. On Day 1, as the blood washes against the hypothalamus and anterior pituitary there is practically no estrogen in it. As a result, the hypothalamus sends a pulse of its hormone GnRH to wake up the pituitary. The receptors on the cells that make up the anterior pituitary gland respond to the rise in GnRH and the lack of estrogen in the bloodstream. Their response is to release FSH into the bloodstream, also in pulses. The presence of FSH in the bloodstream signals to the ovaries and adrenals to start making estrogen.

For the following 10 days of a regular normal cycle, the anterior pituitary gland will be putting out FSH in pulses to stimulate the ovary to make the much-needed estrogen.

Indirectly the pulses of FSH together with the now rising levels of estrogen are responsible for another important job. Remember that FSH stands for follicle stimulating hormone. Its job is to stimulate the formation of the follicle in the ovary and the maturation of an egg that will then be released from the ovary at ovulation.

In the ovary, the egg has been identified. This egg (ovum) will become mature over the following 10 days. It is this egg that will be expelled from the ovary at the time of ovulation, 15 days before the end of the cycle.

It is this egg that if fertilized by a sperm may become a baby 10 months later.

FSH and estrogen help the egg mature to prepare it for ovulation. This part of the cycle is called the follicular phase. The ovary is making estrogen and testosterone to help the egg ripen. Their job is to create a protective bubble around the egg, the follicle, inside which the egg matures. Once mature, the egg and its follicle are expelled from the ovary on ovulation day.

As this scenario unfolds, the increased levels of estrogen produced by the ovary and follicle are now reaching the pituitary and sending a new message to the master gland: "We have enough estrogen here to go ahead and ovulate."

If the pituitary reads the message correctly it starts releasing LH (luteinizing hormone). LH promotes ovulation. Within 10 to 12 hours of the spike of LH in our bloodstream, we ovulate. LH stimulates the production of progesterone, the thinning of the wall of the ovary, the expulsion of the egg from the ovary and the beginning of the luteal phase of the cycle. Once ovulation has occurred, 15 days before the start of the next period, LH levels drop rapidly.

While FSH is around for the better part of the cycle, stimulating the production of estrogen with its attendant effects, LH production is turned off by the increasing levels of progesterone. Progesterone is made by the corpus luteum, the name given to the follicle once expelled (pushed out) from the ovary, now an independent organ responsible for further support and preparation of the egg for fertilization and implantation into the wall of the uterus. Progesterone made by the corpus luteum prevents other eggs from maturing and keeps the uterine lining thick and ready for implantation of the fertilized egg. More than 90 percent of the body's progesterone is made by this short-lived organ. If the woman gets pregnant, the corpus luteum thrives and makes literally gallons of progesterone to nurture and sustain the fertilized egg and then the fetus. If the woman doesn't get pregnant, the corpus luteum shrinks and dies, and progesterone, as well as estrogen, production drop precipitously over the ensuing few days. The cycle has ended and the woman gets her period. The fall of estrogen and progesterone is picked up by the hypothalamus. This signals the start of a new cycle and the hypothalamus heralds it by secreting GnRH again.

The cycle repeats itself every month until we either get pregnant or stop ovulating regularly during perimenopause and totally at menopause and after, surgically or chemically changing the way our bodies function (hysterectomies with oophorectomies, birth control pills and other hormone blockers like Tamoxifen, Evista, and so on).

APPENDIX B

Sex Hormones 101
Estrogen

Estrogen is made in the ovaries, the follicle around the ovum, adrenal glands and fat cells.

Estrogen is not one big molecule; it is a group of molecules. The three main estrogen molecules known are: estriol, estradiol, and estrone.

Estradiol (E2) *es-TRA-di-ol*—Estradiol is the estrogen of youth. It is manufactured by our ovaries, adrenals, and fat cells as we get older and, sometimes, unfortunately fatter. Estradiol directly affects the functions of all our organs. Practically every cell in our body has receptors for estradiol on its cell membrane. This means that estradiol can directly attach to every cell in our body and directly affect its function. Thus, estradiol modifies organ function directly and significantly.

Estriol (E3) *ES-tree-ol*—Estriol is the weakest of estrogens. It is mainly made by the placenta, meaning it is most abundant in our bodies when we are pregnant. In addition to its presence in the placenta it also attaches to cell membrane receptors affecting hair, nails, mucous membranes (vagina), and skin. Data on its function beyond pregnancy point to effects primarily on the vaginal walls and skin but not on the heart, brain or bones. In nonpregnant women, estriol is made in the liver in small doses that cannot be measured with normal laboratory testing. Use of estriol as a supplemental estrogen is limited to skin creams and vaginal creams. Estriol may decrease pore size and increase collagen production in the skin but the scientific data on it is scant at best. Vaginally, using estriol in combination with DHEA (testosterone precursor) may increase vaginal wall thickness, maintain lubrication and increase libido in menopausal women. There is no scientific data to support other usage for it although a drug made of estriol was evaluated by the FDA for use in multiple sclerosis but did not pass the approval process.

Estrone (E1) *es-TRONE*—Estrone is produced after menopause in fat cells primarily from testosterone derivatives (androstenedione, *andro-STENE-di-own*). Estrone is also present in women on birth control pills, perimenopausal, premenopausal, menopausal, and postmenopausal women. Estrone has been implicated in increased incidence of breast tumors. Most data come from animal studies and there is limited knowledge in the medical community about the role of estrone in the aging woman. Overweight older women have high circulating levels of Estrone and so do older men. One European study revealed higher levels of circulating Estrone in women with breast cancer. Using it to supplement hormone regimens is not recommended and preparations containing estrone should not be used (such as Tri-Est, a compounded formulation).

When we refer to estrogen many people refer to all three estrogens as one. At times, this attempt to simplify creates errors in separating their individual actions. The component molecules have different potencies and different outcomes and uses.

For now, let's just remember that when I refer to estrogen in this book, I am referring to what is chemically identified as 17-beta estradiol only, unless otherwise specified.

This molecule, 17-beta estradiol, is the estrogen known under other names including bioidentical, natural, and human identical and is available in compounded forms and FDA-approved formulations.

Starting in our 30s during perimenopause, the production of estrogen by the ovaries diminishes in quantity and quality, leaving much of the work to the adrenal glands and fat cells after menopause. The body transforms unused testosterone into estrogen and calls upon estrogen stored in fat cells as well. The only hormone made after menopause is DHEA, which is a hormone precursor and may or may not metabolize to active hormones. Estrogen and progesterone are antagonists. Their actions are designed to balance each other, to keep each other in check.

As we begin to examine their individual effects keep in mind that at no time do they act independently, under normal circumstances, in healthy bodies. Even creating this list of separate functions for the two hormones leads to confusion at times but many physicians and women want to be able to separate their actions. Thus, I will try to create this artificial separation to help us better understand the role of hormones in wellness and disease prevention.

Estrogen makes everything grow.

The positive effects of its action are that estrogen:

- ▶ Makes the lining of the uterus grow to prepare for pregnancy.
- ▶ Helps the breast tissue grow in preparation for making milk (not in the sense of cancer growth).
- ▶ Causes the ovum to mature inside the ovary to prepare for ovulation.
- ▶ Creates the follicle where the egg matures.
- ▶ Promotes the growth of the fetus in the uterus.

- ▶ Keeps the vagina, vulva, and cervix well-developed and moisturized.
- ▶ Promotes growth of underarm and pubic hair, and pigmentation of the nipples.
- ▶ Stimulates body fat accumulation to prevent starvation of the fetus.
- ▶ Prevents bone destruction by bone-destroying cells (blocks osteoclast action).
- ▶ Protects from heart disease by relaxing the blood vessels and reducing coronary artery contraction that leads to ischemia (not enough blood to the heart muscle).
- ▶ Stimulates the production of lipoprotein lipase, an enzyme that breaks down fat. The result is low cholesterol levels and healthy balance between good (HDL) cholesterol and bad (LDL) cholesterol.
- ▶ Lowers insulin levels.
- ▶ Improves mood by increasing serotonin release in the brain.
- ▶ Helps you sleep by increasing hormone production in the brain, improving quality and quantity of sleep.

The negative effects of estrogen are:

- ▶ Increased accumulation of body fat specifically around the waist.
- ▶ Increased water and salt retention.
- ▶ Interference with normal insulin release and blood sugar control (increased incidence of insulin resistance).
- ▶ Increased risk of overgrowth of endometrium (lining of the uterus).
- ▶ Increased risk of overgrowth of breast tissue.
- ▶ Increased risk of bloating.

▶ Increased risk of headaches.

▶ Increased incidence of irritability.

▶ Increased risk of formation of gallstones.

Progesterone

Progesterone is made primarily by the corpus luteum (the follicle left after ovulation), and is a precursor to most sex hormones. Progesterone levels increase in the middle of the woman's menstrual cycle.

Stimulated by the release of LH (luteinizing hormone) by the pituitary gland in pulses, progesterone is crucial to the survival of the ovum once fertilized. When pregnancy occurs, progesterone production increases rapidly and is taken over by the placenta. If the woman does not get pregnant, the corpus luteum shrinks, progesterone production falters and so does estrogen production. As the hormones leave the system menstruation starts.

Progesterone is the precursor, or parent, of estrogen in the ovaries. Adrenal glands and testes also manufacture it. Progesterone is the precursor of testosterone, all androgens (male hormones) and other adrenal hormones, making it important for reasons far beyond its role as sex hormone.

Progesterone's positive actions are to:

▶ Prepare the endometrium for implantation of the fertilized ovum.

▶ Ensure survival of the fetus in the uterus.

▶ Prevent water retention.

▶ Help use fat for energy at the cellular level.

▶ Serve as a natural antidepressant.

▶ Create a calming effect on the body.

▶ Help improve quality of sleep.

- ▶ Help keep insulin release in check and maintain balanced blood sugar levels.
- ▶ Prevent overgrowth of the endometrium.
- ▶ Prevent breast tissue overgrowth.
- ▶ Maintain sex drive.
- ▶ Maintain normal blood-clotting parameters.
- ▶ Protect against fibrocystic breasts.

Progesterone's negative effects are:

- ▶ Sedation
- ▶ Loss of sex drive
- ▶ Increased spotting
- ▶ Changes in bleeding patterns (either shortening or lengthening menstrual cycle)
- ▶ Bloating from water retention
- ▶ Gastrointestinal discomfort and irritation
- ▶ Acne
- ▶ Hyperpigmentation of facial skin and abdominal striae
- ▶ Headaches

As you can see, the effects of estrogen and progesterone are intermingled and difficult to separate. They often do the same thing so attributing one individual action to one alone is impossible and when treating patients can be even dangerous.

Testosterone

Considered THE male hormone, testosterone is very important in the normal hormone balance of both women and men.

Produced primarily in the testicles and adrenals in men, and in the adrenals, ovaries, and corpus luteum in women, testosterone is part of a larger class of hormones called androgens.

APPENDIX B

These hormones have primarily masculinizing effects. Like estrogens, when we speak of androgens (*ANDRO-gens*), we include more than one hormone: testosterone (*tes-TOS-te-rone*), androstenediol (*andro-STENE-di-ol*), dihydrotestosterone (*DI-hydro-tes-TOS-te-rone*), androstanediol (*andro-STANE-di-ol*), androstenedione (*andro-STENE-di-own*), and dehydroepiandrosterone (DHEA) (*di-HYDRO-epi-andro-STERONE*).

All these hormones are results of the natural breakdown of testosterone and different people are genetically programmed to follow different pathways in the metabolism of testosterone, leading to different quantities of these hormones.

The most widely recognized role for testosterone is the determinant of male characteristics. Although this may seem straightforward and almost too simplistic, testosterone functions are of major significance to women as well.

Testosterone helps to:

- ▶ Promote muscle strength and exercise endurance
- ▶ Improve libido
- ▶ Increase energy levels
- ▶ Improve sense of well-being
- ▶ Increase body hair production
- ▶ Produce enlargement of the penis and testes as well as clitoris
- ▶ Improve sexual desire and fantasy
- ▶ Improve bone density
- ▶ Protect cardiac function
- ▶ Maintain mental acuity
- ▶ Maintain sense of well-being

The negative effects of testosterone are due to overproduction or intake through unsupervised androgen supplementation in pharmaceutical formulations, also known as anabolic steroids.

The NIH states: *"Anabolic steroids is the familiar name for synthetic substances related to the male sex hormones (e.g., testosterone). They promote the growth of skeletal muscle (anabolic effects) and the development of male sexual characteristics (androgenic effects) in both males and females."* Available since the 1930s, these include THG (tetrahydrogestrinone) and androstenedione (andro). The list of commonly abused steroids includes: Anadrol (oxymetholone), Oxandrin (oxandrolone), Dianabol (methandrostenolone), Winstrol (stanozol), Deca-Durabolin (nandrolone decanoate), Durabolin (nandrolone phenylpropionate), and others.

The side-effects may include:

▶ Male pattern baldness
▶ Increased facial hair
▶ Aggressive behavior
▶ Irritability
▶ High cholesterol levels
▶ Clitoral enlargement
▶ Testicular shrinkage
▶ Growth of breast tissue in men
▶ Deepening of voice in both sexes
▶ Acne
▶ Increased number of red blood cells
▶ Decreased sperm count

Please note that anabolic steroids are referred to as *"synthetic substances related to the male sex hormones (e.g., Testosterone)"* by the NIH; they are no different than all the estrogens and progestogens I mentioned in previous paragraphs. If they are not estrogen, progesterone, or testosterone, they are synthetic substances *related to* the male and female sex hormones. Only human identical or bioidentical hormones are the same as the human hormones.

APPENDIX C

IV Intraveonous Infusions

Another important addition to the armamentarium of prevention includes IVs. Removing them from the acute care environment of ERs and hospitals has brought IVs to the public and expanded their use in prevention.

In our practice at Evolved Science, we have been using individualized combinations of fluids, supplements, enzymes, vitamins and other natural substances our bodies require to function optimally. The results have been nothing short of miraculous as our patients, under the supervision of physicians and nurses, receive individualized IV formulations that help:

- ► Improve immune function
- ► Decrease inflammation
- ► Hydrate
- ► Help prevent and shorten the duration of colds and flu
- ► Support hormone function
- ► Increase energy production at the cellular level
- ► Improve recovery and preparation for elective surgeries
- ► Improve body's ability to withstand chemotherapy and radiation toxicity and negative side-effects

▶ Detoxify from anesthesia and other toxicity-laden medical and surgical treatments.

For more on IV infusions, please go to www.eshealth.com or call our offices.

Resources

www.eshealth.com
www.drerika.com
www.bhionline.org
www.medquest.com

Recommended Reading

Female Brain Gone Insane, Mia Lundin

Getting Through Menopause, Haley Lynn

I Just Want to Be ME Again, Jeanne D. Andrus

Menopause: How to Naturally Manage Menopause, Treat Menopause Symptoms With Natural, Holistic Treatments, and Home Remedies, Patricia Pain

Sweetening the Pill, Holly Grigg-Spall

The Hot Topic, Christa D'Souza

The Menopause Thyroid Solution, Mary J. Shomon

The Truth About Men and Sex, Abraham Morgentaler

Testosterone for Life, Abraham Morgentaler

The Viagra Myth, Abraham Morgentaler

The Wisdom of Menopause, Christiane Northrup

You're not Losing Your MIND, You're Losing Your HORMONES!, Sindi J. Holmlund

References

Harman SM, Brinton EA, Cedars M, Lobo R, Manson JE, Merriam GR, Miller VM, Naftolin F, Santoro N. "KEEPS: The Kronos Early Estrogen Prevention Study." *Climacteric.* 2005 Mar;8(1):3-12.

Lippert T, Seeger H, Mueck A. "Pharmacology and toxicology of different estrogens. *G Endodonzia* 2001;15:26–33.

Stanzcyk F. "Estrogen used for replacement therapy in postmenopausal women." *G Endodonzia* 2001;15(4):17–25.

Ribot C, Tremollieres, F. "Hormone replacement therapy in postmenopausal women. All the treatments are not the same." Gynecol Obstet Fertil 2007;35: 1–10.

Schindler A, Campagnoli C, Druckman R, et al. "Classification and pharmacology of progestins." *Maturitas* 2003;46:S7–16.

Smith D, Prentice R, Thompson D, et al. "Association of exogenous estrogen and endometrial carcinoma." *N Engl J Med* 1975;293(23):1164–6.

Ziel H, Finkle W. "Increased risk of endometrial carcinoma among users of conjugated estrogens." *N Engl J Med* 1975;293(23):1167–70.

Stanczyk FZ. "All progestins are not created equal." *Steroids* 2003;68:879–90.

Druckman R. "Progestins and their effects on the breast." *Maturitas* 2003;46: 59–69.

Colditz G. "Estrogen, estrogen plus progestin therapy, and risk of breast cancer." *Clin Cancer Res* 2005;11:909–17.

Callantine M, Martin P, Bolding OT, et al. "Micronined 17b-estradiol for oral estrogen therapy in menopausal women." *The Am Col of Obstet Gynecol* 1975;46: 37–41.

Greenblatt R, Stoddard L. "The estrogen-cancer controversy." *J Am Geriatr Soc* 1978;26(1):1–8.

Whitehead M, Townsend P, Gill D, et al. "Absorption and metabolism of oral progesterone." *BMJ* 1980;280(6217):811–27.

Bergkvist L, Adami H, Persson I, et al. "The risk of breast cancer after estrogen and estrogen-progestin replacement." *NEJM* 1989;321(5):293–7.

Place V, Powers M, Schenkel L, et al. "A double-blind comparative study of estraderm and premarin in the amelioration of postmenopausal symptoms." *Am J Obstet Gynecol* 1985;152(8):1092–9.

Riis B, Thomsen K, Strom V, et al. "The effect of percutaneous estradiol and natural progesterone on postmenopausal bone loss." *Am J Obstet Gynecol* 1987; 156(1):61–5.

Maxson W, Hargrove J. "Bioavailability of oral micronized progesterone." *Fertil Steril* 1985;44(5):622–6.

Whitehead M, Fraser D, Schenkel L, et al. "Transdermal administration of oestrogen/progesterone hormone replacement therapy." *The Lancet* 1990;335: 310–2.

Writing group for the PEPI trial. "Effects of estrogen or estrogen/progestin regimens on heart disease risk factors in postmenopausal women. The postmenopausal estrogen/progestin interventions (PEPI) trial." *JAMA* 1995;273:199–208.

Nelson HD. "Commonly used types of postmenopausal estrogen for treatment of hot flashes." *JAMA* 2004;291(13):1610–20.

References

Fournier A, Berrino F, Riboli E, et al. "Breast cancer risk in relation to different types of hormone replacement therapy in the E3N-EPIC cohort." *Int J Cancer* 2005;114:448–54.

Fournier A, Berrino F, Clavel-Chapelon F. "Unequal risks for breast cancer associated with different hormone replacement therapies: results from the E3N cohort study." *Breast Cancer Res Treat* 2008;107(1):103–11.

Campagnoli C, Abba C, Ambroggio S, et al. "Breast cancer and hormone replacement therapy: putting the risk into perspective." *Gynecol Endocrinol* 2001;15:53–60.

Schindler A. "European Progestin Club. Differential effects of progestins." *Maturitas* 2003;46:S3–5. 2007;14(3):1–6.

Simon JA, Bouchard C, Waldbaum A, et al. "Low dose of transdermal estradiol(E2) gel for treatment of symptomatic postmenopausal women." *Obstet Gynecol* 2007;109(2):1–10.

Zegura B, Guzic-Salobir B, Sebestjen M, et al. "The effect of various menopausal hormone therapies on markers of inflammation, coagulation, fibrinolysis, lipids, and lipoproteins in healthy postmenopausal women." *Menopause* 2006;13(4): 643–50.

Rossow J, Anderson G, Prentice R, et al. Writing Group for the Women's Health Initiative. "Risks and benefits of estrogen plus progestin in healthy postmenopausal women." *JAMA* 2002;288(3):321–33.

Statement on the estrogen plus progestin trial of the Women's Health Initiative. *ACOG* News release 2002.

HERS Study report. "HT can relieve menopause-type symptoms common in elderly women." *ACOG* News Release 2002.

Jernstrom H, Bendahl P, Lidfeldt J, et al. "A prospective study of different types of hormone replacement therapy use and the risk of subsequent breast cancer: the Women's Health in the Lund Area (WHILA) study (Sweden)." *Cancer Causes Control* 2003;14:673–80.

Dobs A, Nguyen T. "Differential effects of oral estrogen versus oral estrogen-androgen replacement therapy on body composition in postmenopausal women." *Clin Endocrinol Metab* 2002;87:1509–16.

Davis S, Davidson S, Donath S. "Circulating androgen levels and self-reported sexual function in women." *JAMA* 2005;294:91–6.

Winters J. "Current status of testosterone replacement therapy in men." *Arch Fam Med* 1999;8:257–63.

Mulligan T, Frick M, Zuraw Q, et al. "Prevalence of hypogonadism in males aged at least 45 years: the HIM study." *Int J Clin Pract* 2006;60(7):762–9.

Shippen E, Fryer W. *The testosterone syndrome: the critical factor for energy, health and sexuality—reversing the male menopause.* New York: M Evans and Company; 1998.

Khaw K, Dowsett M, Folkerd E, et al. "Endogenous testosterone and mortality due to all causes, cardiovascular disease, and cancer in men." European Prospective Investigation into Cancer in Norfolk (EPIC-Norfolk) prospective population study. *Circulation* 2007;116:2694–701.

Shores MM, Matsumoto AM, Sloan KL, et al. "Low serum testosterone and mortality in male veterans." *Arch Intern Med* 2006;166:1660–5.

English KM, Steeds RP, Jones HT, et al. "Low-dose transdermal therapy improves angina theshold in men with chronic stable angina: a randomized, double-blind place-controlled study." *Circulation* 2000;102:1906–11.

Rodriguez A, Muller DC, Metter EJ, et al. "Aging, androgens, and the metabolic syndrome in a longitudinal study of aging." *J Clin Endocrinol Metab* 2007;92(9): 3568–72.

Herbst K, Bhasin S. "Testosterone action on skeletal muscle." *Curr Opin Clin Nutr Metab Care* 2004;7(3):271–7.

References

Shabsigh R, Kaufman J, Steidle C, et al. "Randomized study of testosterone gel as adjunctive therapy to sildenafil in hypogonadal men with erectile dysfunction who do not respond to sildenafil alone." *The Journal of Urology* 2008;179(5): S97–102.

Saad F, Grahl AS, Aversa A, et al. "Effects of testosterone on erectile function: implications for the therapy of erectile dysfunction." *BJU Int* 2007;99(5): 988–92.

Huggins C, Hodges CV. "Studies on prostatic cancer I: the effects of castration, of estrogen and of androgen injection on serum phosphotases in metastatic carcinoma of the prostate." *Cancer Res* 1941;1:293–7.

Huggins C, Stevens RE, Hodges CV. "Studies on prostatic cancer II: the effects of castration on advanced carcinoma of the prostate gland." *Arch Surg* 1941;43: 209–23.

Morgentaler A. "Testosterone replacement therapy and prostate cancer." *Urol Clin North Am* 2007;34:555–63.

Harman S. "Testosterone in older men after the Institute of Medicine report: Where do we go from here?" *Climacteric* 2006;77(5):1319–26.

Travison T, Araujo AB, O'Donnell AB, et al. "A population-level decline in serum testosterone levels in American men." *J Clin Endocrinol Met* 2007;92(1): 196–202.

Matsumoto AM. "Hormonal therapy of male hypogonadism." *Endocrinol Metab Clin North Am* 1994;23:857–75.

Morgentaler A. "Commentary: guidelines for male testosterone therapy: a clinician's perspective." *J Clin Endocrinol Metab*

Canaris GJ, Manowitz NR, Mayor G, et al. "The Colorado thyroid disease prevalence study." *Arch Intern Med* 2000;160:526–34.

Mcdermott MT, Ridgway C. "Subclinical hypothyroidism is mild thyroid failure and should be treated." *J Clin Endocrinol Met* 2001;86(10):4585–90.

Joffe RT, Levitt AJ. "Major depression and subclinical (grade 2) hypothyroidism." *Psychoneuroendocrinology* 1992;17:215–21.

Haggerty JJ Jr, Stern RA, Mason GA, et al. "Subclinical hypothyroidism: a modifiable risk factor for depression?" *Am J Psychiatry* 1993;150(3):508–10.

Manciet G, Dartigues JF, Decamps A, et al. "The PAQUID survey and correlates of subclinical hypothyroidism in elderly community residents in the southwest of France." *Age Ageing* 1995;24:235–41.

Ridgway EC, Cooper DS, Walker H, et al. "Peripheral responses to thyroid hormone before and after L-thyroxine therapy in patients with subclinical hypothyroidism." *J Clin Endocrinol Metab* 1981;53:1238–42.

Tanis BC, Westendorp RGJ, Smelt AHM. "Effect of thyroid substitution on hyper- cholesterolaemia in patients with subclinical hypothyroidism: a re-analysis of intervention studies." *Clin Endocrinol* 1996;44:643–9.

Michalopoulou G, Alevizaki M, Piperingos G, et al. "High serum cholesterol levels in persons with 'high normal' TSH levels: Should one extend the definition of subclinical hypothyroidism." *Eur J Endocrinol* 1998;138:141–5.

Bindels AJ, Westendorp RG, Frolich M, et al. "The prevalence of subclinical hypothyroidism at different total plasma cholesterol levels in middle aged men and women: a need for case-finding?" *Clin Endocrinol* 1999;50:217–20.

Walsh JP, Bremner AP, Bulsara MK, et al. "Subclinical thyroid dysfunction as a risk factor for cardiovascular disease." *Arch Intern Med* 2005;165(21):2467–72.

Docter R, Krenning EP, de Jong M, et al. "The sick euthyroid syndrome: changes in thyroid hormone serum parameters and hormone metabolism." *Clin Endocrinol (Oxf)* 1993;39:499–518.

Chopra IJ. "Euthyroid sick syndrome: Is it a misnomer?" *J Clin Endocrinol Metab* 1997;82(2):329–34.

References

Kok P, Roelfsema F, Langendonk JG, et al. "High circulating thyrotropin levels in obese women are reduced after body weight loss induced by caloric restriction." *J Clin Endocrinol Metab* 2005;90:4659–63.

Mariotti S, Barbesino G, Caturegli P, et al. "Complex alterations of thyroid function in healthy centenarians." *J Clin Endocrinol Met* 1993;77(5):1130–4.

Pingitore A, Galli E, Barison A, et al. "Acute effects of triiodothyronine replacement therapy in patients with chronic heart failure and low T3 syndrome: a randomized placebo-controlled study." *J Clin Endocrinol Met* 2008;93:1351–8.

Smidt-Ott UM, Ascheim DD. "Thyroid hormone and heart failure." *Curr Heart Fail Rep* 2006;3:114–9.

Carle A, Laurberg P, Pedersen IB, et al. "Thyrotropin secretion decreases with age in patients with hypothyroidism." *Clinical Thyroidology* 2007;17:139–44.

van den Beld AW, Visser TJ, Feelders RA, et al. "Thyroid hormone concentrations, disease, physical function and mortality in elderly men." *J Clin Endocrinol Metab* 2005;90(12):6403–9.

Hermann J, Heinen E, Kroll HJ, et al. "Thyroid function and thyroid hormone metabolism in elderly people low T3–syndrome in old age." *Klin Wochenschr* 1981; 59:315–23.

Fukagawa NK, Bandini LG, Young JB. "Effect of age on body composition and resting metabolic rate." *Am J Physiol Endocrinol Metab* 1990;259:E233–8.

van Coevorden A, Laurent E, Decoster C, et al. "Decreased basal and stimulated thyrotropin secretion in healthy elderly men." *J Clin Endocrinol Metab* 1989;69: 177–85.

Rubenstein HA, Butler VPJ, Werner SC. "Progressive decrease in serum triiodothyronine concentrations with human aging: radioimmunoassay following extraction of serum." *J Clin Endocrinol Metab* 1973;37:247–53.

Chakraborti S, Chakraborti T, Mandal M, et al. "Hypothalamic–pituitary–thyroid axis status of humans during development of ageing process." *Clin Chim Acta* 1999;288(1-2):137–45.

Piers LS, Soars MJ, McCormack LM, et al. "Is there evidence for an age-related reduction in metabolic rate?" *J Appl Phys* 1998;85:2196–204.

Poehlman ET, Berke EM, Joseph JR, et al. "Influence of aerobic capacity, body composition, and thyroid hormones on the age-related decline in resting metabolic rate." *Metabolism* 1992;41:915–21.

Magri F, Fioravanti CM, vignati G, et al. "Thyroid function in old and very old healthy subjects." *J Endocrinol Invest* 2002;25(10):60–3. *Hormones in Wellness and Disease Prevention* 705

Goichot B, Schlienger JL, Grunenberger F, et al. "Thyroid hormone status and nutrient intake in the free-living elderly. Interest of reverse triiodothyronine assessment." *Eur J Endocrinol* 1994;130:244–52.

Cizza G, Brady LS, Calogero AE, et al. "Central hypothyroidism is associated with advanced age in male Fischer 344/n rats: in vivo and in vitro studies." *Endocrinology* 1992;131:2672–80.

American College of Sports Medicine (ACSM) Fit Society Page. Available at: http:// www.acsm.org/AM/Template.cfm?Section About_ACSM&CONTENTID13519& TEMPLATE/CM/ ContentDisplay.cfm. Accessed March 20, 2011.

ABOUT THE AUTHOR

Dr. Erika Schwartz is an internationally renowned thought leader and pioneer in the field of prevention, patient centered healthcare, hormone balance, lifestyles, and supplements. Her work integrates body and mind treatments using all modalities. Dr. Erika's groundbreaking book *Don't Let Your Doctor Kill You* exposed the truth about our flawed health care system and empowered patients to take control over their own healthcare.

Combining a Renaissance European upbringing, American education, passion for the patient, kindness, and common sense, Dr. Erika is the founder and Medical Director of Evolved Science, a concierge medical practice in New York City focused on exceptional and respectful patient services. Dr. Schwartz received her undergraduate degree with honors from New York University, and her MD from SUNY-Downstate College of Medicine, Cum Laude. She is a member of Alpha Omega Alpha honor society and past president of the Board of Managers.

Dr. Erika is world renowned for her expertise and leadership in the conventional use of bioidentical hormones for women and men; supplements; patient advocacy; integration of diet, exercise, and lifestyle; stress and relationship management; and spiritual growth in all patient care. She is a firm believer the doctor's role of serving the patient and the crucial importance of patient-centric healthcare must be measured in excellent outcomes. She lives in New York City.